ACADEMIC HEALTH CENTERS

Leading Change in the 21st Century

Committee on the Roles of Academic Health Centers in the 21st Century
Linda T. Kohn, Editor

INSTITUTE OF MEDICINE
OF THE NATIONAL ACADEMIES

THE NATIONAL ACADEMIES PRESS
Washington, D.C.
www.nap.edu

THE NATIONAL ACADEMIES PRESS • 500 Fifth Street, N.W. • Washington, DC 20001

NOTICE: The project that is the subject of this report was approved by the Governing Board of the National Research Council, whose members are drawn from the councils of the National Academy of Sciences, the National Academy of Engineering, and the Institute of Medicine. The members of the committee responsible for the report were chosen for their special competences and with regard for appropriate balance.

This study was supported by Contract No. 01-267 and 20010609 between the National Academy of Sciences and The Rockefeller Brothers Fund, with additional support from The Commonwealth Fund, the Institute of Medicine, and the National Research Foundation. Any opinions, findings, conclusions, or recommendations expressed in this publication are those of the author(s) and do not necessarily reflect the view of the organizations or agencies that provided support for this project.

Library of Congress Cataloging-in-Publication Data

Academic health centers : leading change in the 21st century / Committee on the Roles of Academic Health Centers in the 21st Century ; Linda T. Kohn, editor.
   p. ; cm.
Includes bibliographical references and index.
ISBN 0-309-08893-3 (hardcover)
1. Academic medical centers—United States.
   [DNLM: 1. Academic Medical Centers—trends—United States. WX 27 AA1 A168 2004] I. Kohn, Linda T. II. Institute of Medicine (U.S.). Committee on the Roles of Academic Health Centers in the 21st Century.
RA966.A23 2004
362.12—dc22
                           2004001871

Additional copies of this report are available from the National Academies Press, 500 Fifth Street, N.W., Lockbox 285, Washington, DC 20055; (800) 624-6242 or (202) 334-3313 (in the Washington metropolitan area); Internet, http://www.nap.edu.

For more information about the Institute of Medicine, visit the IOM home page at: www.iom.edu.

Copyright 2004 by the National Academy of Sciences. All rights reserved.

Printed in the United States of America.

The serpent has been a symbol of long life, healing, and knowledge among almost all cultures and religions since the beginning of recorded history. The serpent adopted as a logotype by the Institute of Medicine is a relief carving from ancient Greece, now held by the Staatliche Museen in Berlin.

*"Knowing is not enough; we must apply.
Willing is not enough; we must do."*
—Goethe

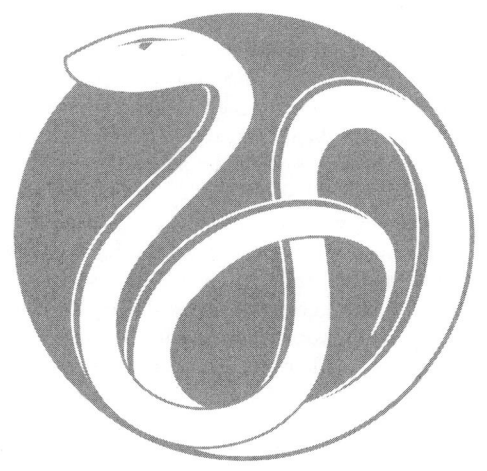

INSTITUTE OF MEDICINE
OF THE NATIONAL ACADEMIES

Adviser to the Nation to Improve Health

THE NATIONAL ACADEMIES
Advisers to the Nation on Science, Engineering, and Medicine

The **National Academy of Sciences** is a private, nonprofit, self-perpetuating society of distinguished scholars engaged in scientific and engineering research, dedicated to the furtherance of science and technology and to their use for the general welfare. Upon the authority of the charter granted to it by the Congress in 1863, the Academy has a mandate that requires it to advise the federal government on scientific and technical matters. Dr. Bruce M. Alberts is president of the National Academy of Sciences.

The **National Academy of Engineering** was established in 1964, under the charter of the National Academy of Sciences, as a parallel organization of outstanding engineers. It is autonomous in its administration and in the selection of its members, sharing with the National Academy of Sciences the responsibility for advising the federal government. The National Academy of Engineering also sponsors engineering programs aimed at meeting national needs, encourages education and research, and recognizes the superior achievements of engineers. Dr. Wm. A. Wulf is president of the National Academy of Engineering.

The **Institute of Medicine** was established in 1970 by the National Academy of Sciences to secure the services of eminent members of appropriate professions in the examination of policy matters pertaining to the health of the public. The Institute acts under the responsibility given to the National Academy of Sciences by its congressional charter to be an adviser to the federal government and, upon its own initiative, to identify issues of medical care, research, and education. Dr. Harvey V. Fineberg is president of the Institute of Medicine.

The **National Research Council** was organized by the National Academy of Sciences in 1916 to associate the broad community of science and technology with the Academy's purposes of furthering knowledge and advising the federal government. Functioning in accordance with general policies determined by the Academy, the Council has become the principal operating agency of both the National Academy of Sciences and the National Academy of Engineering in providing services to the government, the public, and the scientific and engineering communities. The Council is administered jointly by both Academies and the Institute of Medicine. Dr. Bruce M. Alberts and Dr. Wm. A. Wulf are chair and vice chair, respectively, of the National Research Council.

www.national-academies.org

COMMITTEE ON THE ROLES OF ACADEMIC HEALTH CENTERS IN THE 21ST CENTURY

The Honorable JOHN EDWARD PORTER (*Chair*), Partner, Hogan and Hartson, L.L.P. Washington, DC, Member of Congress 1980-2001

LINDA AIKEN, Claire M. Fagin Professor of Nursing and Sociology and Director, Center for Health Outcomes and Policy Research, University of Pennsylvania, Philadelphia, Pennsylvania

J. CLAUDE BENNETT, President and Chief Operating Officer, BioCryst Pharmaceuticals, Inc., Birmingham, Alabama

HENRY BIENEN, President, Northwestern University, Evanston and Chicago, Illinois

NANCY-ANN MIN DEPARLE, Adjunct Professor of Health Care Systems, Wharton School, University of Pennsylvania; Senior Adviser, JP Morgan Partners, New York, New York

EDWARD W. HOLMES, Vice Chancellor for Health Sciences and Dean, University of California San Diego School of Medicine, La Jolla, California

LAWRENCE LEWIN, Executive Consultant, Washington, D.C.

NICOLE LURIE, Senior Scientist and Alcoa Professor of Policy Analysis, The RAND Corporation, Arlington, Virginia

STEVEN M. PAUL, Group Vice President, Lilly Research Laboratories, Eli Lilly Company, Indianapolis, Indiana

PAUL G. RAMSEY, Vice President Medical Affairs and Dean, University of Washington School of Medicine, Seattle, Washington

ROBERT REISCHAUER, President, The Urban Institute, Washington, DC

JOHN W. ROWE, Chairman and CEO, Aetna Inc., Hartford, Connecticut

MARLA SALMON, Dean and Professor, Nell Hodgson Woodruff School of Nursing, Emory University, Atlanta, Georgia

CHRISTINE SEIDMAN, Howard Hughes Medical Institute and Brigham and Women's Hospital, Professor of Medicine and Genetics, Harvard Medical School, Boston, Massachusetts

M. ROY WILSON, President, Texas Tech University Health Sciences Center, Lubbock, Texas. Until June 2003, Dean, School of Medicine and Vice President for Health Sciences, Creighton University, Omaha, Nebraska

LIAISON FROM THE BOARD ON HEALTH SCIENCES POLICY

JAMES CURRAN, Dean and Professor of Epidemiology, Rollins School of Public Health, Emory University, Atlanta, Georgia

STUDY STAFF

LINDA T. KOHN, Study Director
MARYANN BOLCAR, Program Officer
RANDA KHOURY, Project Assistant
RONNÉ D. WINGATE, Project Assistant
JANET M. CORRIGAN, Director, Board on Health Care Services

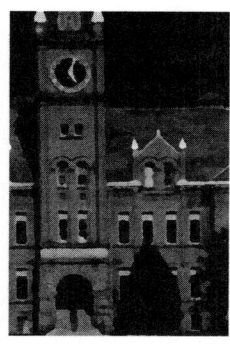

REVIEWERS

This report has been reviewed in draft form by individuals chosen for their diverse perspectives and technical expertise, in accordance with procedures approved by the NRC's Report Review Committee. The purpose of this independent review is to provide candid and critical comments that will assist the institution in making its published report as sound as possible and to ensure that the report meets institutional standards for objectivity, evidence, and responsiveness to the study charge. The review comments and draft manuscript remain confidential to protect the integrity of the deliberative process. We wish to thank the following individuals for their review of this report:

Henry Aaron, Brookings Institution, Washington, DC
David Blumenthal, Massachusetts General Hospital, Partners Healthcare, Boston, Massachusetts
David R. Challoner, University of Florida, Gainesville, Florida
Don E. Detmer, Cambridge University Health, Judge Institute of Management, Cambridge, UK
Robert Galvin, General Electric Company, Fairfield, Connecticut
Harry R. Jacobson, Vanderbilt University, Nashville, Tennessee
Peter O. Kohler, Oregon Health & Sciences University, Portland, Oregon
Ronda Kotelchuck, Primary Care Development Corporation, New York, New York

Joel Kupersmith, Texas Tech University, Lubbock, Texas
Mary O. Mundinger, Columbia University, New York, New York
Cecil B. Pickett, Schering-Plough Research Institute, Kenilworth, New Jersey
Mitchell T. Rabkin, Harvard University, Cambridge, Massachusetts
Leon E. Rosenberg, Princeton University, Princeton, New Jersey
Linda Rosenstock, University of California, Los Angeles
Bruce Vladeck, Mt. Sinai School of Medicine, New York, New York

Although the reviewers listed above have provided many constructive comments and suggestions, they were not asked to endorse the conclusions or recommendations nor did they see the final draft of the report before its release. The review of this report was overseen by **Robert Johnson, Professor, New Jersey Medical School**, appointed by the Institute of Medicine, and **Enriqueta Bond, President, Burroughs Wellcome Fund**, appointed by the National Research Council. They were responsible for making certain that an independent examination of this report was carried out in accordance with institutional procedures and that all review comments were carefully considered. Responsibility for the final content of this report rests entirely with the authoring committee and the institution.

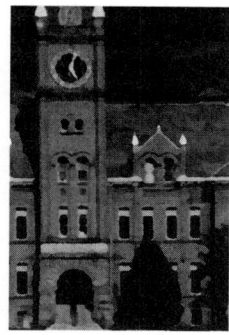

Preface

The last few decades have been heady times for science and health. Our knowledge of how to improve health has grown significantly and new technologies have successfully supported those endeavors. The coming decades are likely to bring even more progress. As we gain a better understanding on how to use the discoveries of genetics, proteomics, and other biologies, we will have the potential to fundamentally alter care in ways that we can only begin to imagine. Combined with a public that is armed with more information and better able to make healthy choices and be more involved in its own care, the potential is great for making large strides in improving human health.

In the fall of 2001, the Institute of Medicine convened a committee to examine the roles of academic health centers (AHCs) in the coming decades in fostering and supporting these advances in health care. The challenge to this committee was to look into the future and consider how AHCs can be prepared to fulfill their promise by carrying out their roles in education, research, and patient care to improve health for all people. AHCs demonstrated great vision and accomplishment during the 20th century. They will need these qualities in the coming decades if they are to adapt and respond to the changing needs of people and the expanding capabilities that health care will offer.

This committee was intentionally designed to include a diverse group of individuals from varied backgrounds so as to bring contrasting views to the subject at hand. The members did not always agree, and on occasion a dissenting voice even rose, reflecting the seriousness with which the members viewed their charge. By the end of the deliberations, a mutual respect had grown for the always thoughtful views expressed by each committee member. I am thankful for the opportunity to work with such an experienced, visionary, and talented group. Excellent staff support was also provided by Maryann Bolcar, Ronne Wingate, and Randa Khoury, under the able and patient direction of Linda Kohn.

The challenges facing AHCs in the future will be significant. Change is never easy and rarely smooth. But the opportunities are too great to forsake. I speak for the entire committee in believing that strong AHC leadership and sound policy support will indeed make it possible to achieve better health for all.

John Edward Porter
Chair
June 2003

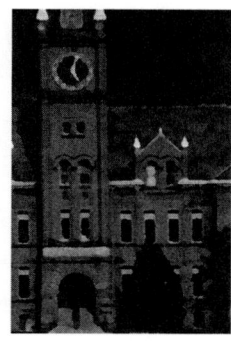

Acknowledgments

The Committee on the Roles of Academic Health Centers in the 21st Century gratefully acknowledges the contributions of the many individuals and organizations through the course of the study that participated and gave generously of their time and knowledge.

Support for this study was provided by the Institute of Medicine, the National Research Council, the Rockefeller Brothers Foundation, and The Commonwealth Fund. The Committee especially recognizes Melinda Abrams of The Commonwealth Fund, and Linda Jacobs and William McCalpin of the Rockefeller Brothers Foundation, for their special attention to this project.

A workshop was sponsored by the committee in January 2002 during which the following people offered their views on the future roles for AHCs: Gerard Anderson, Johns Hopkins University; Brian Biles, George Washington University; Joseph D. Bloom, Oregon Health and Science University; David Blumenthal, Partners HealthCare System; Samuel Broder, Celera Genomics; Jordan Cohen, Association of American Medical Colleges; Colleen Conway-Welch, Vanderbilt University; Charles Cutler, American Association of Health Plans; Ezra Davidson, Charles R. Drew University; Robert Dickler, Association of American Medical Colleges; Gerald Fischbach, Columbia University; Jeff Goldsmith, Health Futures Inc.; Ralph Horwitz, Yale University; Edward Hundert, Case Western Reserve University; Darrell Kirch, Pennsylvania State University; Uwe E. Reinhardt, Princeton University; Sara Rosenbaum, George Washington

University; Elaine Rubin, Association of Academic Health Centers; Ralph Snyderman, Duke University; and Bruce C. Vladeck, Mount Sinai School of Medicine.

Several university presidents made presentations about their own AHCs. The committee is grateful to Lee C. Bollinger of Columbia University, Judith Rodin of the University of Pennsylvania, Leonard W. Sandridge of the University of Virginia, and Stephen J. Trachtenberg of the George Washington University for sharing their knowledge. In addition, Catherine Dower of the University of California, San Francisco, and Robert Galvin of General Electric provided valuable testimony to the Committee during a July 2002 meeting.

The Committee acknowledges with gratitude a number of others for providing their time and expertise to this work: Helene Bednash, American Association of Colleges of Nursing; Linda Berlin, American Association of Colleges of Nursing; Roger Bulger, Association of Academic Health Centers; Molly Cooke, University of California San Francisco; Alain Enthoven, Stanford University; The Honorable Bill Gradison, Patton Boggs; David Helms, AcademyHealth; George Kaludis, Kaludis Consulting; Brian Kimes, National Cancer Institute; Peter Kohler, Oregon Health and Science University; Jay Levine, ECG Management Consultants; Craig Lisk, Medicare Payment Advisory Commission; Alexander Omaya, Institute of Medicine; Marian Osterweis, Association of Academic Health Centers; Julian Pettingill, Medicare Payment Advisory Commission; James Reuter, Georgetown University; Edward Salsberg, University of Albany SUNY; Ellen Stovall, National Coalition for Cancer Survivorship; and Linda Weiss, National Cancer Institute.

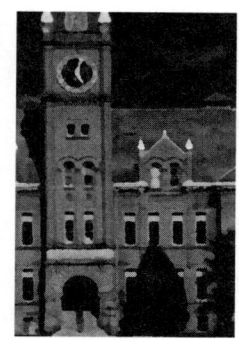

CONTENTS

EXECUTIVE SUMMARY   1

1   INTRODUCTION   19

2   FORCES FOR CHANGE   30

TRANSFORMING THE ROLES OF AHCS

3   THE ACADEMIC HEALTH CENTER AS A REFORMER:
    THE EDUCATION ROLE   45

4   THE ACADEMIC HEALTH CENTER AS A MODELER:
    THE PATIENT CARE ROLE   65

5   THE ACADEMIC HEALTH CENTER AS A TRANSLATOR
    OF SCIENCE: THE RESEARCH ROLE   77

CREATING AN ENVIRONMENT FOR INNOVATION

6   THE CONSEQUENCES OF CURRENT FINANCING
    METHODS FOR THE FUTURE ROLES OF AHCs   92

7	EXPECTATIONS FOR THE AHC OF THE 21ST CENTURY	110
8	CREATING SYSTEMS FOR CHANGE IN AHCs	127
	REFERENCES	144

APPENDIXES

A	ACADEMIC HEALTH CENTERS: ALL THE SAME, ALL DIFFERENT, OR ...	161
B	COMMITTEE ON THE ROLES OF ACADEMIC HEALTH CENTERS IN THE 21ST CENTURY	198

Executive Summary

ABSTRACT

The Committee on the Roles of Academic Health Centers in the 21st Century convened in November 2001 with the charge of examining the current role and status of academic health centers (AHCs) in American society; anticipating intermediate and long-term opportunities and challenges for AHCs; and recommending to the AHCs themselves, to policy makers, to the health professions, and to the public, scenarios that might be undertaken to maximize the public good associated with these institutions.

Technological, demographic, social, and economic trends will have a significant impact on the roles performed by AHCs. The committee believes that changes will be required in each of those roles if AHCs are to continue to meet the public's needs in the coming decades. To this end, the external environment should create a set of incentives that will clearly signal the need for change and serve as a spur for actions by AHCs. In the area of education, Congress should create a dedicated fund that can support efforts to foster innovation in the methods and approaches used to prepare health professionals; in response, AHCs will need to examine fundamentally the methods and approaches used to prepare health professionals. In the area of research, federal funding agencies should work together to support collaborations by a mix of scien-

tists who do different types of research to answer the important questions of science and health; in response, AHCs will need to examine how their research programs link across the continuum of research. In the area of patient care, public and private payers and foundations should support experimentation in working across settings of care to redesign and restructure care processes aimed at improving the health of both patients and populations; in response, AHCs will need to create the structures and team approaches needed to focus on health for patients and populations.

Accomplishing these changes will require that AHCs establish the strategic management systems necessary to create an environment for innovation and enable a more coordinated and cohesive systemwide view across the multiple roles and organizations represented in each AHC. These systems include improved information systems, mechanisms for accountability to measure and reward progress in meeting AHC-wide goals, and leadership development and support. As each AHC makes its own decisions on how to respond to its changing environment, it should recognize the interdependent and complementary nature of the AHCs' traditionally individual roles within an overall context and commitment to improving the health of the American people.

While academic health centers (AHCs) have made important contributions to the health of people in this nation and internationally, there is no question that the future will present a very different set of demands on these institutions. Biomedical and other technological advances are creating a constantly expanding knowledge base that must be harnessed and applied if its benefits are to be realized. Concepts of medicine, health, and preventive care will be fundamentally redefined as knowledge from research on the human genome and other new scientific endeavors offer new treatments and the ability to customize care to meet individual needs and characteristics. More so than acute illness, chronic conditions are now the leading cause of illness, disability, and death and account for the majority of health resources used today (Hoffman, et al., 1996; Foundation for Accountability and The Robert Wood Johnson Foundation, 2002), they are greatly influenced by people's lifestyles and personal choices, opening the door for a lifelong, more integrative view of health. Information and telecommunications technology is a major force in cultivating a more informed consumer and can engage patients in exerting more direction and control over their care, altering their interactions with and expectations from clinicians. Expanding technology and knowledge also provide opportunities for the health care system to achieve goals of much higher levels of quality and safety.

Moreover, health care, like all industries, is affected by globalization that speeds the transfer of knowledge, but also the transmission of disease.

AHCs face significant challenges in addressing these developments. They are large and complex organizations that make available a broad and complex set of services, and function in a dual safety net role, serving the most severely ill as well as many poor and uninsured. They are concerned about the disruption of traditional funding streams brought about by marketplace competition and about being placed at a disadvantage because of their higher costs due to their education and research roles. But the challenges that confront AHCs as a result of the trends noted above are not purely market driven, nor are they temporary. They represent fundamental and long-term technological, demographic, and social shifts that will force AHCs to examine what they do and how they carry out their various roles.

AHCs must respond to their changing environment. The choices they make have an effect well beyond their own organizations, influencing the capabilities that reside throughout the health system generally and the kind of health care the American people will enjoy. Decisions about how to train health professionals influence the clinical skills they use in practicing within the larger system. Decisions about what types of research to pursue and how to share the results influence future practice patterns and insurance policies. Additionally, AHCs receive a significant level of public support for their activities. Over the last decade, the federal and state governments have allocated approximately $100 billion to support activities in clinical education and research, as well as disproportionate-share funds to care for the poor and uninsured (Anderson, 2002). Much of this funding has gone to support the activities of AHCs, so the nation has the right to look to them for guidance and leadership in addressing the health needs of the American people.

For this report, the committee views an AHC not as a single institution, but as a constellation of functions and organizations committed to improving the health of patients and populations through the integration of their roles in research, education, and patient care to produce the knowledge and evidence base that become the foundation for both treating illness and improving health. Although AHCs vary in their organization and the emphasis placed on these roles, the committee believes they all face similar challenges.

Before offering its recommendations, the committee wishes to emphasize its serious concern regarding the problems facing people who are uninsured, recognizing the relationship among a lack of insurance, difficulties in accessing care, and an individual's health (Institute of Medicine, 2001a, 2002). In addition to the health impacts on uninsured individuals and populations, AHCs that care for a disproportionate share of the poor and uninsured bear a financial burden that may affect their ability to continue to carry out their core activities in research and education. The committee has not made a specific recommendation regarding this problem because its impact is broader than AHCs. However, we strongly urge that the ranks of the uninsured be reduced, and that AHCs devote more of their attention to the future challenges of improving the health and well-being of all people.

RECOMMENDATIONS

The committee offers a relatively small number of recommendations that together form a two-part strategy. The overall strategy aims to initiate a continuing and long-term process of change. First, the external environment should create a set of incentives that will clearly signal the need for change in each of the AHC roles and serve as a spur for actions by AHCs. In the area of education, Congress should create a dedicated fund that can support efforts to foster innovation in the methods and approaches used to prepare health professionals; in response, AHCs will need to examine fundamentally the methods and approaches used to prepare health professionals. In the area of research, federal funding agencies should work together to support collaborations by a mix of scientists doing different types of research to answer the important questions of science and health; in response, AHCs will need to examine how their research programs link across the continuum of research. In the area of patient care, public and private payers and foundations should support experimentation in working across settings of care to redesign and restructure care processes aimed at improving the health of both patients and populations; in response, AHCs will need to create the structures and team approaches needed to focus on health for patients and populations.

AHCs will not be able to take up the challenge of making the changes called for in each role with minor adaptations or a focus on each role in isolation from the others. Adding one more course to an already overcrowded curriculum or doing one more research study will not be sufficient. Furthermore, because of the interdependence of the AHC roles, changes in one role affect the others. For example, improving the educational experience for students involves much more than curricular reform, also requiring changes in the practice setting in which students are taught. Similarly, no one component of an AHC can make the changes recommended. A school can modify its own curriculum but cannot unilaterally impose more interdisciplinary approaches.

Therefore, the second part of our proposed strategy addresses the AHCs themselves, asking them to examine how they organize, perform, assess, and internally support their various roles. Our recommendations call on

AHCs to establish systems across all of their organizations and roles to facilitate the flow of information throughout the AHC, establish and measure AHC-wide goals for change, and develop and support leaders who will take on the transformations required.

In developing such systems, AHCs will need to recognize the interdependent and complementary nature of their traditionally individual roles within an overall context that encompasses a commitment to improving the health of patients and populations. Indeed, the unique contribution of AHCs in the coming decades will lie in their ability to achieve such an integration of their roles within medicine and across all health sciences, including public health, nursing, dentistry, pharmacy, and others, to foster the health of all Americans. This integration involves more than the simultaneous provision of education, research, and patient care. It requires the purposeful linkage of these roles so that research develops the evidence base, patient care applies and refines the evidence base, and education teaches evidence-based and team-based approaches to care and prevention.

Transforming the Roles of AHCs for the 21st Century

Reforming the Education of Health Professionals

AHCs have historically emphasized the education of physicians at the undergraduate and graduate levels, relying on the hospital's inpatient and outpatient settings as primary training sites. To respond to the changing needs of the population and the changing demands of practice in the 21st century, AHCs will have to play a leading role in the transformation of education for all health professionals.

Recommendation 1:

AHCs should take the lead in reforming the content and methods of health professions education to include the integrated development of educational curricula and approaches that:

a. Enable and encourage coordination among deans of various professional schools and leaders across disciplines (such as medicine, dentistry, nursing, public health, pharmacy, social work, and basic sciences) to remove internal barriers to interprofessional education.

b. Ensure that all teaching environments—from the classroom to sites for clinical rotations and preceptorships and practice—are exemplars for the future of health care delivery (e.g., by modeling team-based care and using information technology) and, in collaboration with local health care leaders, demonstrate how to improve health for populations and communities, as well as individual patients.

c. Emphasize training in skills that will be needed to improve health, such as the theory and computational skills necessary to comprehend the new biological sciences, as well as the social and behavioral sciences.

d. Develop, recognize and reward those who teach and conduct research on clinical education.

Health care practitioners will not be prepared for practice in the 21st century without fundamental changes in the approaches, methods, and settings used for all levels of clinical education. Current training of health professionals emphasizes primarily the biological basis of disease and treatment of symptoms, with insufficient attention to the social, behavioral, and other factors that contribute to healing and are part of creating healthy populations. The training of disciplines in separate "silos" creates boundaries where coordination and collaboration are needed to improve health. Furthermore, there is little coordination among undergraduate, graduate, and continuing education; the result is duplication in some areas and gaps in others.

Health professions training is a major factor in creating the culture and attitudes that will guide a lifetime of practice. For most health professionals, more than half their training occurs in clinical settings rather than the classroom. The clinical setting in which students are trained must be able to demonstrate care that is patient-centered and health-improving, and to model practices that are evidence-based, continuously improving, and cost-efficient. New approaches to clinical education will be required, especially to reflect practice in interdisciplinary teams and greater use of information and communications systems.

AHCs should take a lead role in reforming clinical education. Education oversight organizations (accrediting, licensing, and certifying bodies) should also work together to revise their standards, as recommended in a recent Institute of Medicine (2003a) report that calls for an overhaul in health professions education. In addition, funders should send a clear signal that reform in health professions education is important and must happen more quickly.

Recommendation 2:

Congress should support innovation in clinical education through changes in the financing of clinical education.

a. Congress should create an ongoing fund that provides competitive grants to support educational innovation.

- Funds should support educational innovations such as use of clinical information systems, testing of new educational approaches in hospital and nonhospital settings, and evaluation of curricular and other needed reforms in clinical education. Priority for such funds should be given to those organizations that integrate the training of multiple health disciplines (e.g., medicine, nursing, pharmacy, therapy, public health, administration) and that use information technology in their clinical education programs.

- To create this education innovation fund, Congress should redirect the portion of the funding provided for indirect medical education that exceeds the additional costs of caring for Medicare patients that are attributable to teaching activities (commonly referred to as the "empirical amount"). Availability of these funds should be contingent upon implementing innovations in clinical education and training environments.

b. In addition, Congress and the Administration should promptly revise the current statutory framework of Medicare support for graduate medical education to support more interdisciplinary, team-based, nonhospital training that aims to improve the health of patients and populations. Revisions should include consideration of whether other payers should provide specific support for the education of health professionals; examine the relationship between support for the training of physician and nonphysician clinicians; assess the appropriate recipient of support; and identify mechanisms for accountability for both the disbursement and the use of public funds.

The committee recommends a two-pronged approach to address both short- and long-term issues in the financing of clinical education. First, the recommended innovation fund should be created using a portion of the public resources currently devoted to existing programs to initiate immediate change in individual training programs. AHCs need to make changes in the content, methods, and approaches for clinical education, and support should be provided for those efforts through the innovation fund. Second, more broad-based, long-lasting changes are also needed. The committee does not question continued support for health professions education, but we believe that current methods are insufficient to support future needs and should be fundamentally revised to encourage the training of a workforce that will be prepared to work in the interdisciplinary, health-oriented, information-driven models of care of the 21st century.

The committee identified three options for creating an education innovation fund. One was to create a new funding program. The education of health professionals is of sufficient value to society to justify the allocation of new funds to such an endeavor. Another option was to freeze current payments for graduate medical education and channel the inflationary adjustment that would occur under the existing program into the innovation fund. Using this mechanism, about $40 million would have been made available to such a fund in 2001.[1] The third option was to redirect a portion of the current funding for indirect medical education (IME) to support reforms in clinical education.

IME payments to teaching hospitals are intended to support the additional costs of caring for Medicare patients that are attributable to teaching activities. Analyses by the Medicare Payment Advisory Commission (MedPAC) revealed that Medicare's IME adjustment formula for 2002 is about twice the calculated estimate of these higher costs (Medicare Payment Advisory Commission, 2002). For 2003, MedPAC estimates that about 2.5 percentage points of the 5.5 percent IME add-on (about $2.6 billion) is in excess of the current cost relationship (Medicare Payment Advisory Commission, 2003). In its March 2003 Report to Congress, MedPAC expressed its dissatisfaction with current payment methods that provide no accountability for the use of funds beyond the Medicare payment amount related to increased patient care costs in teaching hospitals (Medicare Payment Advisory Commission, 2003).

The committee does not deem it likely that an entirely new funding source could be created, and does not believe that redirecting the increment provided by inflation would provide sufficient funds to support the endeavor. Using a portion of the IME add-on would produce a larger pool of funds to support educational innovation.

The committee believes that as the primary funder of graduate medical education, Medicare has a responsibility to send a clear signal on the need for change in these programs to ensure the availability of an adequately prepared workforce that is able to meet the health needs of the Medicare population. Furthermore, as noted previously, making the types of changes in clinical education suggested here will affect patient care. It can be assumed, therefore, that those changes will also affect the costs of treating Medicare patients in teaching hospitals, which is the intended purpose of providing the IME percentage add-on.

It is important to recognize that the committee does not recommend a reduction of overall support to AHCs. Rather, our recommendation directs

---

[1] This figure assumes that $2 billion was provided to hospitals for direct medical education costs and that the Consumer Price Index was 2 percent.

that AHCs have the opportunity to retain the funds and that Medicare have the opportunity to send a strong signal for change while inserting a level of accountability for the use of those funds. Although the recommendation does not represent a loss of funds to AHCs, it could represent a loss of flexibility in their use. For example, to the extent that an AHC uses IME funds to subsidize care to the uninsured, there is a risk that such services could be curtailed.[2] The Centers for Medicare and Medicaid Services and MedPAC should carefully monitor the effects of the establishment of the innovation fund for any deleterious effects.

Although the proposed innovation fund can provide an incentive for immediate change, current funding methods for clinical education do not adequately support training in nonhospital settings, foster interdisciplinary approaches to training, or consider the relationship between the training of physician and nonphysician clinicians. Current methods have encouraged growth in the number, size, and duration of medical residency programs and the training of specialists in inpatient tertiary settings (Henderson, 2000; Young and Coffman, 1998). For nurses and allied health professionals (including, for example, physician assistants), current payment methods have favored programs in settings that do not train physicians and are not linked to universities. Current policies do not give either AHCs or Medicare the flexibility or encouragement to make adjustments as workforce needs change, even when clear needs are identified, such as clinicians to care for an aging, chronically ill population. State and federal policy makers continue to struggle with persistent problems regarding the mix and distribution of health professionals. Work on revising the current statutory framework to address these issues should proceed promptly while the innovation fund helps spur immediate changes.

Demonstrating New Models of Care

Changing health needs and changing technologies create both demands and opportunities for new models of care that are designed to improve health.

Recommendation 3:

AHCs should design and assess new structures and approaches for patient care.

---

[2]This is an example that could be true for some hospitals, but not others as research shows a weak relationship between the hospitals that receive IME funds and the hospitals that serve the most poor and uninsured (Medicare Payment Advisory Commission, 2003; Anderson et al., 2001).

a. AHCs should work across disciplines and, where appropriate, across settings of care in their communities to develop organizational structures and team approaches designed to improve health. Such approaches should be incorporated into clinical education to teach health-oriented processes of care.

b. Public and private payers, state and federal agencies, and foundations should provide support for demonstration projects designed to test and evaluate the organizational structures and team approaches designed to improve health and prevent disease. Demonstrations should target in particular (1) populations that are at high risk for serious illness, (2) populations that are financially vulnerable, (3) conditions that reflect disparities across the population, and (4) methods for supporting individuals' involvement in and decisions about their health. Demonstrations should encompass both financing and delivery components, including the testing of organizational reforms that optimize work design and workforce management. Payers should streamline the process for incorporating successful demonstration results into coverage and payment policies.

As the health needs of people change and the health care system's capabilities expand, the potential to improve health will grow. There is clearly room for improving processes of care to impact health, as has been demonstrated for chronically ill populations, for the frail elderly, and for uninsured populations (Institute of Medicine, 2001b; Wagner et al., 1996; Bodenheimer et al., 2002; Wieland et al., 2000; Kaufman et al., 2000). AHCs should be part of efforts to conceptualize new models of care and communicate to payers and policy makers the characteristics of care models that can improve the health of patients and populations that are at high risk for serious illness and those that are financially vulnerable since these populations are especially reliant on AHCs. AHCs are well positioned to demonstrate new models of care because of the intersection of patient care with their other roles. As AHCs develop the evidence base, it can be applied in patient care and demonstrate to students good patterns of practice.

Developing structures and approaches that can improve the health of both patients and populations will require AHCs to examine critically the processes of care within their own care settings, and reach out to their surrounding communities to collaborate with other providers and services (including complementary and alternative health services) and with public health agencies. Within their own setting, AHCs will need to examine how to improve systems of service and care to make them safer and more effective and efficient, particularly as technological advances permit new ways of designing work. The changing composition of the health care workforce, combined with shortages in some areas, will require that models of care improve not only quality, but also productivity. AHCs should be using their patient care settings to test organizational reforms that can optimize work design and workforce management (including evidence-based management), thereby increasing retention of health professionals and reducing dissatisfaction with the work environment.

To encourage and support innovations aimed at redesigning care to improve health, public payers (such as the Centers for Medicare and Medicaid Services and state Medicaid programs) and private payers (such as insurance companies and managed care organizations) need to support innovations in both financing and delivery so payers can use the results and facilitate their replication in other practice settings. Payment policy is a strong influence on how care is designed and delivered, and for the most part, current payment methods do not provide sufficient recognition or reward for improving health or quality or preventing disease (Institute of Medicine, 2001).

Translating the Discoveries of Science into Improved Health

AHCs have been significant contributors to the enormous strides made in research in recent years. The challenge in the coming decades will be to apply those advances and new laboratory discoveries to clinical settings and community practices so their benefits will reach more people.

Recommendation 4:

Health-related research needs to span the continuum from discovery to testing to application and evaluation.

a. AHCs should increase their emphasis on clinical, health services, prevention, community-based, and translational research that can move basic discoveries into clinical and community settings.

b. Congress and the administration should coordinate funding across agencies that support health-related research including the life sciences (biomedical, clinical, health services, and prevention research), the physical sciences, and other sciences that advance health. More coordinated funding efforts and the criteria for evaluating funding support should foster interdisciplinary and collaborative arrangements that cut across departments, professional schools, and institutions.

Historically, AHCs have focused on basic biomedical research, with support from the National Institutes of Health. They have emphasized in particular basic scientific research, a foundation for the health-related "research and development" activities that make future advances possible. It is important to maintain strong support for such research to sustain continued scientific advances; however, the coming decades will require an increased emphasis on clinical, health services, and prevention research to translate the discoveries of basic science into clinical and community practice and to improve health. Research should be aimed at answering questions in a variety of areas, such as the clinical, organizational, and cost effectiveness of new therapies as well as current practices to assess what does and does not work in health care; effective methods for promoting healthy behaviors; the design of safe, efficient, and effective processes of care that are able to blend personal and preventive health practices; and methods for incorporating best practices into various clinical settings. Greater priority should also be given to how organizations can translate the findings of health services research into institutional and other settings.

Asking AHCs to consider research across the continuum does not mean asking every AHC to expand its research activities. Rather, each should strategically assess its resources and capabilities to set priorities for how those resources can be applied to improve health, and to determine how it can establish and reward the collaborative, interdisciplinary approaches that characterize clinical, health services, and prevention research, and support the types of collaborations needed for translating discoveries into practice. For example, applying the knowledge of genetics to care will require not only basic research to understand the mechanisms involved, but also clinical and prevention research to apply results to care, attention to issues of organizational design so providers can deliver the care, an understanding of costs and financing to build use of that knowledge into the health system, and a focus on how to educate patients and professionals so everyone understands the potential and limitations of the resulting care. Yet each of these matters is addressed by different scientists who are funded separately, and usually by different agencies.

At the federal level, health-related research is funded by the National Institutes of Health, the Centers for Disease Control and Prevention, the Health Resources and Services Administration, the Agency for Healthcare Research and Quality, the Centers for Medicare and Medicaid Services, the Food and Drug Administration, the Veterans Health Administration, the Department of Defense, the Department of Energy, the Environmental Protection Agency, the National Science Foundation, and even the National Aeronautics and Space Administration (National Science and Technology Council, 2000). One example of funding for collaborative efforts has been support for research centers, such as the cancer centers program at the National Cancer Institute which funds interdisciplinary centers conducting research across the continuum that includes basic, clinical, and preventative/behavioral/population-based research (National Cancer Institute, 2002).

Although some interagency funding efforts are in place, improved communication and coordination around funding programs and criteria for both programmatic and training support are needed to facilitate bringing biologists, chemists, physicists, engineers, and mathematicians together with clinical and other investigators, as well as behavioral and social scientists, communication specialists, and others from throughout medicine and public health.

Creating Systems for Change Within AHCs

The recommendations of this report cannot be accomplished simply by adding to the activities of current faculty and organizations, or by making minor adaptations in each AHC role. Rather, clear priorities and decisions will be necessary at the level of the overall AHC, not just its individual organizations. Because of the variability among AHCs, the committee cannot offer a simple prescription for change that would fit all. Instead, we identify several strategic management systems that will be required by all AHCs to create an infrastructure through which to develop an AHC-wide view and systems approach for change across the institution's constellation of roles and organizations.

Utilizing Information and Communications Technology

Information and communications technology is central to the ability of AHCs to perform their roles in the future. It is important, therefore, that AHCs make the implementation of information systems a high priority.

Recommendation 5:

AHCs must make innovation in and implementation of information technology a priority for both managing the enterprise and conducting their integrated teaching, research, and clinical activities.

   a. AHCs should have information systems that span the enterprise for integrated decision making, performance assessment, and financial management.

   b. AHCs need to pioneer the use of information systems for clinical purposes and incorporate their use into clinical education and research.

Information and communications technology is central to all of the roles of AHCs. Basic biomedical research is becoming increasingly reliant on such technology. Emerging areas, such as genomics and proteomics, are based on manipulating large amounts of data. Clinical and health services research, central to translating the results of basic research into clinical care, demand information systems for analysis, synthesis, and dissemination of information. Information technology is important to clinical education as a teaching tool to provide interactive learning models, as well as a way for students to learn to practice in settings that make extensive use of advanced clinical information systems. Moreover, delivery of care and surveillance of health at a population-wide or subgroup level will rely increasingly on good information systems. Finally, information and communications technology are mandatory for managing complex organizations such as AHCs to support accountability for programmatic, strategic, and financial performance.

More broadly, information and communications technology is required to develop the capacity to manage the knowledge and information used and produced by AHCs. Knowledge management has clear clinical applications (including, for example, access to internal and external databases, sharing of best practices, and synthesized updates of developing knowledge), as well as all the knowledge that is useful and/or essential to the proper management of institutions, teams, departments, and interdisciplinary efforts for conducting clinical care, research, and education (The Blue Ridge Academic Health Group, 2000). Therefore, this recommendation requires that the various components of the AHC initiate (or aggressively continue) discussions about creating the capacity for knowledge management and breaking down the barriers that inhibit the sharing of information and knowledge across the organizations and roles of the AHC.

AHCs need to make the implementation of information and communications technology a higher priority. Indeed, capital for such technology needs to be as high a priority as capital for new buildings and equipment. If resources for the purpose are not sufficient within AHCs, federal and state governments should consider ways to encourage the needed investments, particularly for those AHCs that face persistent financial difficulties as a result of serving as safety-net institutions in their communities. Ongoing efforts related to standards and privacy also need to move forward rapidly so that AHCs (and others) can plan and implement their information systems more quickly. The committee urges the development of national data standards to facilitate the development of information and communications technology in health and its incorporation into practice, as well as interoperability of systems and comparability of data (Institute of Medicine, 2003).

Establishing and Measuring AHC-wide Goals for Change

Given the magnitude of the changes required by AHCs, it is important that clear goals be set so that progress toward making those changes can be steadily measured.

Recommendation 6:

Both AHCs and the public should evaluate the progress of AHCs in: (1) redesigning the content and methods of clinical education; (2) developing organizational structures and team approaches in care to improve health; and (3) increasing emphasis on health services, clinical, prevention, and translational research.

a. To aid AHCs in evaluating their progress, the secretary of Health and Human Services should:

- Identify broad areas of AHC performance (e.g., quality of education programs, financial accountability).
- Establish an advisory group to suggest guidelines for measurement and examples of measures that could be used by AHCs.
- Obtain information from AHCs related to the broad areas of performance and issue a report every 2 years on progress made in transforming the roles, identifying areas of success as well as obstacles encountered.

b. University leaders and/or AHC boards of trustees should establish mechanisms for accountability and transparency that can be used to assess their progress toward meeting the goals established for transforming the roles of AHCs.

Because of the functional and organizational variability of AHCs, the committee believes each AHC will need to determine its own goals and priorities, but all will need to create the structures and processes required to support AHC-wide goals and measure their achievement. AHCs will need to look across their entire enterprise to align programmatic, strategic, and financial management; understand the flow of funds; and reorient internal planning and financing arrangements to improve coordination across clinical departments and institutions.

AHCs have traditionally focused on achieving excellence within each of their roles or organizational units, and generally do not set or measure accomplishment of such goals for the AHC enterprise (Zelman et al., 1999; The Commonwealth Task Force on Academic Health Centers, 2000a). While acceptable in stable times, making major change requires a strategic, systemwide view and coordination (Zelman el al., 1999). The challenge is that AHCs are highly complex at both the management and governance levels. Department chairs have traditionally played a very strong role in raising funds, directing budgets, controlling faculty promotion, designing and directing graduate and undergraduate medical education programs, and serving as the liaison between faculty and administration (Bulger, 1988).

The departmental structure is a key element in how an AHC functions, but can also make it difficult to build consensus around AHC-wide goals and priorities. Governance structures can vary as well. An AHC board may have oversight of the medical school but not the nursing school; it may contract with several affiliated hospitals but not own one; or there may not be an oversight board for the AHC itself, only for the individual components.

AHCs will be required to make decisions at the level of the overall AHC and reallocate resources to meet explicit goals for change. Greater transparency, especially in understanding the real financial resources within the AHC and the flow of funds among schools, hospitals, practice plans, and the university, will be required throughout the AHC enterprise, however it is organized.

The Secretary of Health and Human Services can support such efforts by identifying key dimensions of performance and sample measures for each. This work should be done with input from AHCs, states, and groups that rely on the work of AHCs (e.g., employers that hire their trainees). The information should be designed to be useful at both the federal and the state levels.

Leadership for Strategic Change Throughout the AHC

Various models and approaches for undertaking major organizational change have been proposed (Kotter, 1996; Kaplan and Norton, 1996; Plsek, 2001). All emphasize the importance of having a clear vision and strategy for moving forward, and the need for creating the conditions in which change can happen and be rewarded. Organizational change does not just happen; it requires sound leadership at all levels—leadership that should be unambiguously developed, empowered, and supported.

Meeting the challenges set forth in this report will require strong leaders at all levels of the AHC. It will be necessary to establish processes for developing AHC leaders and leadership teams that will be prepared to guide their organizations in the coming decades.

Recommendation 7:

AHCs must be leaders and develop leaders, at all levels, who can:

a. Manage the organizational and systems changes necessary to improve health through innovation in health professions education, patient care, and research.

b. Improve integration and foster cooperation within and across the AHC enterprise.

c. Improve health by providing guidance on pressing societal problems, such as reduction of health disparities, responses to bioterrorism, or ethical issues that arise in health care, research and education.

To accomplish the changes set forth in this report, AHC leaders will need to demonstrate a depth and breadth of leadership unlike anything seen in the past. A major role of leadership is to adapt organizations to changing circumstances (Kotter, 1996). Leadership defines the future, aligns people with a vision, and removes obstacles to realizing that vision. The stakes are high. If AHC leaders at all levels do not have the capabilities required to deliver the results asked of them, the AHCs will not be able to effect the needed changes regardless of how generous the support they receive may be. AHCs will therefore need to invest in programs and processes for identifying, preparing, and developing leaders who can generate and direct the innovations recommended in this report.

In addition to leadership within their own organizations, AHCs need to demonstrate strong leadership to guide the nation toward improved health. They need to speak loudly and clearly for the actions necessary to improve the health of the public, including, for example, the provision of health insurance for all Americans. Meeting this need may be a challenge in that some actions that would improve health may not benefit a specific AHC; for example, better models of care may reduce inpatient admissions, resulting in negative financial consequences for an AHC's hospital. However, maintaining the trust that the country has placed in AHCs requires that they speak out for the nation's health.

In summary, the committee recognizes the vital role that AHCs have played to date, but has asked whether they are appropriately oriented, organized, and financed to meet societal demands for leadership in health. Our conclusion is that absent significant changes in orientation, organization, and both internal and external financing, AHCs may not succeed in fulfilling these expectations. Helping AHCs to meet the challenges of the 21st century will require public policy support, but AHCs must also embark on a period of critical self-evaluation and direct the enormous intellectual energy they house toward leading change in the 21st century.

CHAPTER 1

Introduction

In the fall of 2001, the Institute of Medicine appointed a study committee to examine the roles of academic health centers (AHCs) in the coming decades. While AHCs have made important contributions to health[1] through their combined roles in education, research, and patient care,[2] the future will present a very different set of demands on those roles. The aging of the population is shifting the burden of disease from acute to chronic care. Continued advances in biomedical and information technology will essentially redefine our concepts of medicine and health. Concerns regarding the rising costs of health care, evidence of quality gaps, and worries for many about access to care continue to challenge the health care system.

The goal of this committee was to consider how the environment in which health care is provided is changing, what those changes mean for future demands on the health care system, and implications for how AHCs will carry out their roles in the future to continue to serve the public interest. Other studies of AHCs have generally examined the challenges they face and the implications for the future. Rather than starting with the AHCs themselves, this committee began with the developments and trends occurring in the external environment, focusing on the roles and activities

---

[1]The term *health* is used broadly here to include both health and health care.
[2]Patient care includes care for all people, including the poor and uninsured and other vulnerable groups.

19

performed by AHCs rather than the institutions themselves. This is not a study of clinical education or research or patient care, nor does it focus primarily on any specific organizational component of the AHC, such as a professional school or teaching hospital. Rather, the focus is on the AHC itself and how it will carry out those roles in the future.

Definition of an Academic Health Center

There is no generally accepted definition of an AHC (Anderson et al., 1994). According to the Association of Academic Health Centers, an AHC consists of an allopathic or osteopathic medical school, at least one other health professions school or program, and at least one affiliated or owned teaching hospital (Association of Academic Health Centers, 2002a). The work of the Commonwealth Task Force on Academic Health Centers represents one of the most comprehensive analyses undertaken to better understand the functions of AHCs. That task force defined an AHC as the medical school and its affiliated or owned clinical facilities (The Commonwealth Fund Task Force on Academic Health Centers, 2002). The Association of American Medical Colleges does not explicitly define an AHC, but focuses its efforts on medical schools and their teaching hospitals.

These definitions of an AHC typically start from its organizational components, which consist most commonly of a medical school, other health professions schools (e.g., nursing, pharmacy), and a clinical enterprise. However, the committee recognizes that the organization of AHCs has and will continue to evolve, as it should, and we do not wish to limit their definition to any particular organizational form, especially since the changing environment and demands made on AHCs will likely foster innovative organizational arrangements in the coming years. For example, all AHCs have an owned or affiliated clinical enterprise. In today's environment, the clinical enterprise is most often a hospital, but in the future, it may not have an institutional or hospital base. Similarly, an AHC that is committed to improving the health of patients and populations will be urged to establish relationships and integrate its activities with multiple professional schools, forging linkages through common ownership under a single university or through some other arrangement. Regardless of how the components of any given AHC are assembled, however, the challenges faced will be similar.

For this report, the committee views an AHC not as a single institution, but as a constellation of functions and organizations committed to improving the health of patients and populations through the integration of their roles in research, education, and patient care to produce the knowledge and evidence base that become the foundation for both treating illness and improving health. The core of the AHC constellation is its academic or university-related roles in education and research, which, in combination with patient care, are ultimately aimed at improving the health of people. Because the committee has defined an AHC by its purpose and function, this report focuses on the roles and responsibilities of AHCs rather than their organizational components.

A BRIEF DESCRIPTION OF AHCS

As noted in the definition presented above, today's AHCs link several functions and responsibilities. These linkages came about through a series of events during the 20th century that together produced the AHC we recognize today. First, the Flexner Report of 1910 called for reform of medical education to include a 4-year curriculum comprising 2 years of basic sciences and 2 years of clinical teaching; university affiliation (instead of proprietary schools); requirements for entrance to medical schools; encouragement of active learning, with limited use of lectures and learning by memorization; and emphasis on problem solving and critical thinking (Regan-Smith, 1998; Ludmerer, 1999). By the 1920s, medical education at the hospital bedside had become mandatory (Rosenberg, 1987). Second, during World War II, the federal government increased funding to university research laboratories as a means of supporting the war effort (Korn, 1996). Funding expanded after the war, and increased funding from the National Institutes of Health (NIH) provided support to individual researchers at universities, a pattern that continues today. Third, the passage of Medicare and Medicaid in 1965 ensured revenues for a significant portion of patient care services that had historically been provided as charity care to patients who also helped students learn (Ludmerer, 1999). Significantly, the Medicare program also included support for graduate medical education (Korn, 1996).

The result of these three events is that AHCs found a steady revenue stream for their primary activities and were able to grow their enterprise during the decades that followed (Korn, 1996). Between 1960 and 2000, the U.S. population grew by 54 percent (Centers for Disease Control and Prevention, 2002). During the same period, the number of medical school graduates grew by about 120 percent, the number of basic science faculty grew by more than 330 percent, and the number of clinical faculty grew by more than 1,000 percent (The Commonwealth Fund Task Force on Academic Health Centers, 1997b, 2002). Total funding support from the NIH to medical schools grew by more than 1,500 percent between 1970 and 2000 (National Institutes of Health, 2001). The AHC, as recognized today, then, is a relatively young organization that developed mainly in the latter half of the 20th century.

AHCs have provided important benefits to both local communities and the nation, benefits that accrue to diverse population groups. According to The Commonwealth Task Force on Academic Health Centers, AHCs represent only 3 percent of nonfederal, acute care hospitals in the United States; however, they:

- Care for almost one-third of uninsured patients in their hospitals (The Commonwealth Fund Task Force on Academic Health Centers, 1997a).
- Account for a significant share of the nation's specialized services, such as burn units, transplant programs, and neonatal units (see Appendix A).
- Account for almost one-third of national health-related research and development funds (The Commonwealth Fund Task Force on Academic Health Centers, 1999).
- Produce approximately 16,000 medical school graduates and are the dominant providers of graduate medical education (GME), sponsoring 58 percent of all GME programs (The Commonwealth Fund Task Force on Academic Health Centers, 1997a).
- Graduate about 15,000 nursing school graduates (American Association of Colleges of Nursing, 2002). Each year, almost 40 percent of these graduates are prepared at the master's and doctoral levels, representing an important supply of faculty for all nursing schools (American Association of Colleges of Nursing, 2002).
- Graduate about 6,000 public health professionals annually (Association of Schools of Public Health, 2001).

AHCs also contribute to their local economies. One medium-sized AHC estimated an economic impact on its region of $3.05 billion in a single year through the direct and indirect generation of jobs and spending in its local area (University of Cincinnati Medical Center, 2002). It is estimated that funding from extramural grants by NIH, much of which goes to AHCs, was responsible for providing more than 330,000 jobs in 1999 (Association of American Universities, 2000). Additionally, the development of biomedical campuses by private industry often occurs around AHCs, as in Baltimore and San Diego, for example.

Just over half of AHCs are publicly sponsored organizations; the remainder are private (Osterweis, 1999). Most AHCs are located in urban areas, although a few are rural. AHCs vary in the emphasis placed on each of their roles (see Appendix A). The greatest variation among AHCs is in the size of their research endeavors, in particular, the amount of support they receive from NIH. AHCs also vary in how they combine their roles. One analysis examining the amount of overlap among the top 100 hospitals engaged in teaching, the top 100 hospitals engaged in research, and the top 100 hospitals serving low-income patients revealed that only 25 AHCs rank in the top 100 for all three activities. Of the top 100 hospitals serving low-income patients, 53 are *not* among the top 100 hospitals in education or research (Anderson, et al., 2001).

AHCs comprise many different organizational components. First, all AHCs have a medical school, at a minimum. For some AHCs, that is the only professional school they sponsor; however, the majority of medical schools are located on campuses that have multiple health professions schools and also train nurses, public health or allied health professionals. Second, all AHCs contain one or more hospitals. Third, AHCs also typically have faculty practice plans. These are organizations that focus on delivery of care, and provide a mechanism for structuring a financial relationship between the medical or nursing school and the hospital and between the clinical departments and their clinical faculty (Cohen and Fox, 2003; Rimar, 2000). Most faculty practice plans were developed over the last decade, and their organization and functions continue to evolve. Some AHCs may also have separate research centers (Magill et al., 1998).

These various organizational components come together to form an AHC in a variety of ways. The various components can be independent entities linked together contractually. Alternatively, all the components can come under a single ownership umbrella. A number of AHCs fall in between these two forms, with two of the three components coming under common ownership and contracting with the third component. Organizational variation is also found in the AHCs' governance structure. Individual components may have their own governing boards (which may or may not be linked through coordinating committees), or a single governing board may oversee the entire AHC enterprise. It is not known how many AHCs operate under various forms. Most are loosely affiliated arrangements, with each entity having considerable independence and autonomy (Norlin, et al., 1998). In many cases, the AHC functions rather like a holding company (Zelman, et al., 1999).

Support for the activities of AHCs is not provided to the AHC itself, but goes to its individual components to support specific activities. Support for research generally comes from grants or other programs funded by private industry as well as public agencies, predominantly NIH. Most of these funds go to the medical or other professional school. Support for educational activities and patient care services goes the AHC hospital(s). Support for the direct costs of graduate medical education is provided predominantly by Medicare and some Medicaid programs, as well as special payments, that are made to support the higher patient care costs associated with the sponsorship of training programs. Support for patient care is provided through direct payment for services, as well as special payments from public payers to support care for a disproportionate share of poor and uninsured patients. Private payers usually do not differentiate their support for specific AHC activities, but support the various activities through higher prices paid to AHCs for patient care. Within the AHC, funds are disbursed through a complex arrangement of cross-subsidies to support the particular mix of activities undertaken. For most AHCs, revenues from patient care activities subsidize activities in research and education (The Commonwealth Fund Task Force on Academic Health Centers, 1997b). Funding issues are discussed in greater detail in Chapter 6 of this report.

The committee believes the variability that currently exists among AHCs is likely to continue into the future. The advantage of this situation is the potential for AHCs to respond to varying local demands and to collectively provide a breadth of resources for the nation. This variability, however, created a unique challenge for the committee. Few data are available on the AHCs overall. Information can be obtained about the activities of an AHC hospital or medical school, for example, but there is no data source that provides an overall picture of the AHC enterprise. In conducting its analysis and considering its recommendations, the committee had to recognize that any single prescription would be unlikely to fit all AHCs. At the same time, the committee needed to lay out a future vision and broad direction that would be relevant for all AHCs.

As noted earlier, the committee chose to focus on the roles performed by AHCs and how they fit together, rather than the AHCs' organizational components. Furthermore, the committee chose to focus on how trends in the external environment (as outlined in the next section) will alter expectations for the overall AHC enterprise in the coming decades, rather than on the current pressures facing on the individual AHC organizations. The committee sought further to balance a recognition of the contributions made by AHCs in the past with an emphasis on the demands that will require change in the future.

STUDY FRAMEWORK

The framework for this study assumes that a set of factors in the external environment affects the expectations and demands placed on the health care system overall (see Figure 1-1). These external factors are varied, but the strongest of them can be grouped under three broad categories: (1) people's health care needs are changing as a result of the aging of the population and other demographic developments; (2) technology, including both information and biomedical technologies, is advancing rapidly; and (3) the organization and financing of health care are evolving.

These external factors affect people's health needs and their expectations for the health care system, as well as the capabilities of the system. As the population ages, the burden of disease shifts from acute to chronic illness, and as technology advances, peoples' expectations rise. In addition,

Environmental Changes

People are changing
- Disease burden
- Demographics and labor

Technology is advancing
- Biomedical advances
- Information technology

Organization and financing of care are evolving
- Increasing costs
- Quality concerns
- Size of uninsured population

Public Needs and System Capabilities

Services people need; preferences and expectations

What the system can offer

Care Delivery

What care is provided

How care is provided

Who provides the care

Where the care is provided

AHC Roles

Education

Care for patients and populations

Research

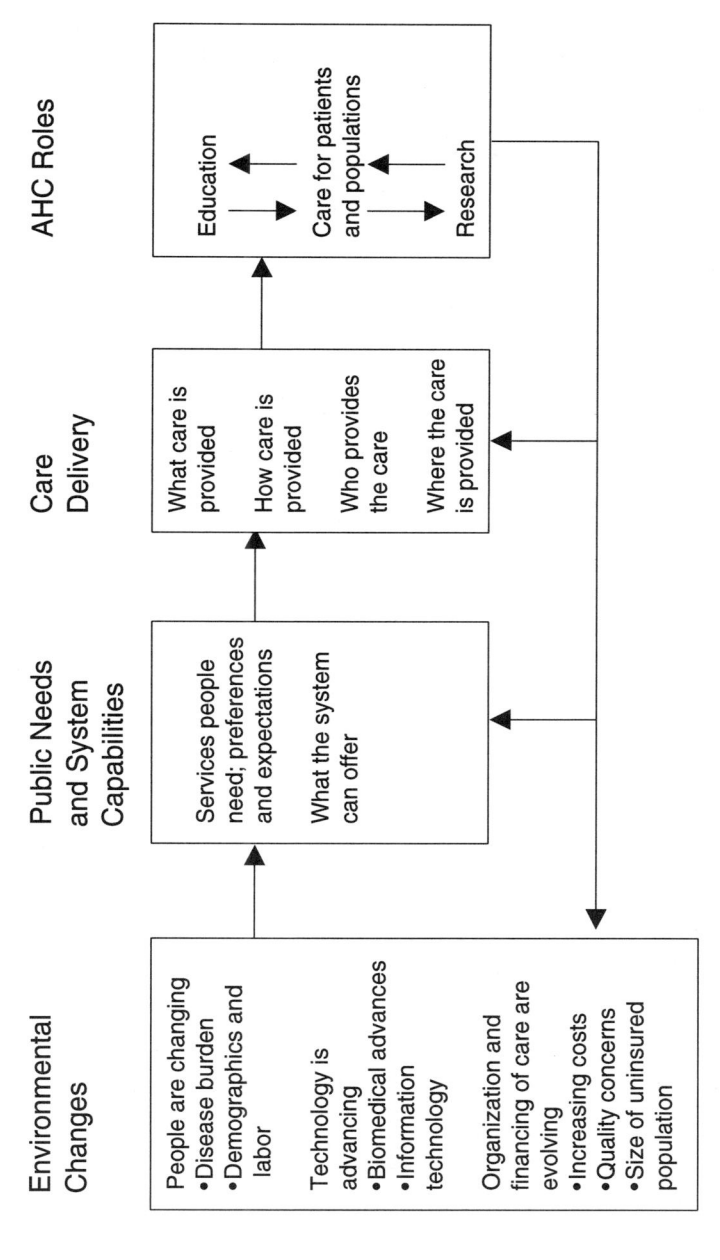

FIGURE 1-1 The Changing Roles of AHCs.

technological advances, combined with changes in the organization and financing of care, provide the health system with additional capabilities. These changing needs, expectations, and capabilities have their most direct impact on care delivery—what care is provided, how it is provided, by whom, and where. For example, services that used to be provided only in a hospital are now offered in ambulatory settings. Likewise, services that may have been provided only by a physician may now be provided by nurse practitioners or nurse anesthetists. The pressures on care delivery ultimately affect the AHC roles in education, research, and patient care. The care provided by AHCs also changes, and as that happens, health professionals must be prepared differently, and research inevitably seeks to answer new questions.

While external forces ultimately affect how AHCs carry out their roles, the actions of AHCs also affect care delivery and peoples' needs and expectations, and even interact with other factors in the external environment (see Figure 1-1). The circular flow of the figure illustrates that AHCs can interact with the external environment in both reactive and proactive ways. For example, information technology affects how health professionals should be trained for practice, but as health professionals receive more training that incorporates information technology, changes can occur in clinical care that affect future training needs. Similarly, genomics is expected to have a significant impact on the care delivered to patients, and health professionals must therefore be trained to deliver the new forms of care. At the same time, as health professionals learn more about the field and gain more experience in applying the science of genomics to people, the care they deliver will also evolve.

STUDY PROCESS

The committee's statement of task is presented in Box 1-1. The committee held six meetings during the course of the study. One meeting was a 2-day workshop at which input was received from AHC leadership, representatives of key constituents served by AHCs (e.g., patients, low-income populations, health plans), and experts in health policy and financing. The workshop agenda is presented in Appendix B. The proceedings of this workshop were published separately and are available at www.nap.edu/catalog/10383.html.

The committee also heard from a number of experts at its other meetings. Leaders from several universities, varying in size, ownership, and organizational structure, offered their views on the risks and rewards of sponsoring an AHC. Presentations were made by Judith Rodin, president, University of Pennsylvania; Lee Bollinger, president, Columbia University (formerly president, University of Michigan); Leonard Sandridge, executive

> **BOX 1-1**
> **Committee Statement of Task**
>
> This study will examine the current role and status of academic health centers in American society, anticipate intermediate and long-term opportunities and challenges for these institutions, and recommend to the institutions themselves, to policy makers, to the health professions, and to the public scenarios that might be undertaken to maximize the public good associated with these institutions.
>
> The committee will:
>
> (1) Assess the development, contribution, and performance of AHCs in teaching, research, and technology development, patient care including the provision of specialized care, and community service including caring for underserved populations.
>
> (2) Evaluate whether AHCs are prepared to meet societal needs and expectations over the coming decades in the areas of a) an educated and trained professional work force; b) assessment of the value and cost effectiveness of new technologies and facilitation of their dispersion; c) provision of health care services to populations dependent upon them (e.g., uninsured, poor); and d) provision of leadership in relation to ethical and social aspects of health.
>
> (3) Assess the capacity of AHCs to carry out their multiple functions in an effective and efficient manner.
>
> (4) Identify steps that can be taken by AHCs themselves, and by communities, policy makers, and others to maintain and enhance the performance of AHCs.

vice president, University of Virginia; and Stephen Joel Trachtenberg, president, George Washington University.

Bill Gradison, vice chair of The Commonwealth Fund Task Force on Academic Health Centers, provided his perspective on the policy issues facing AHCs in the future. Robert Galvin from General Electric provided the committee with a perspective on managing large, complex, and diversified organizations. Catherine Dower of the Center for Health Professions, University of California, San Francisco, discussed with the committee how the workforce is changing generally, as well as within the domain of health care.

The committee relied on a variety of sources for data on the status of AHCs. Requested data were provided by the Association of Academic Health Centers, the Association of American Medical Colleges, and the American Association of Colleges of Nursing. Gerard Anderson of Johns Hopkins University, Bloomberg School of Public Health, conducted an analysis of the extent of variation among AHCs on selected dimensions of their activities in education, research, and patient care. The tables he provided to the committee during its deliberations are included in Appendix A.

The committee also received an analysis conducted by Bruce Steinwald[3] on alternatives for financing the activities of AHCs. His analysis formed the basis for Chapter 6 of this report. Finally, the committee was able to take advantage of information produced by The Commonwealth Task Force on Academic Health Centers. All of its reports that contained recommendations were provided to the committee for reference, serving as a body of knowledge that enabled the committee to conduct its work efficiently without duplicating previous efforts.

The work of this committee was funded through the generous support of The Rockefeller Brothers Fund, with additional support from The Commonwealth Fund, the Institute of Medicine, and the National Research Council.

ORGANIZATION OF THE REPORT

As noted earlier, this report starts not with the AHCs themselves, but with the trends and developments in health care that will affect AHCs in the years ahead. In Chapter 2, the key forces driving these changes are described. This review is followed by chapters examining in turn each of the main roles performed by AHCs, including the status of those activities and the challenges the AHCs will face in carrying out that role in the future. In Chapter 3, the education role is examined, with attention to the approaches used today to educate health professionals for practice tomorrow. Of the three roles performed by AHCs, the education role is expected to face the most profound changes in the coming decades. In Chapter 4, the patient care role is examined, with emphasis on the organizational innovation needed to create better models and approaches for care and to design care around an explicit goal of improving health. In Chapter 5, the research role is examined, with a focus on the importance of spanning the continuum of research—including basic, clinical, health services, and prevention research—to make it possible to translate research findings into practice. Chapter 6 examines how the AHC roles are currently financed and whether those approaches will be able to support the types of changes that will be needed in the future. Chapter 7 synthesizes the information from the prior chapters to offer a set of recommendations for transforming the roles of AHCs to meet the challenges of the changing environment of health care. Chapter 8 considers the management and leadership challenges facing AHCs as they contend with having to undergo that transformation.

---

[3]At the time that Mr. Steinwald prepared the analysis for the committee, he was working as an independent consultant.

Each of the topics considered by the committee could have been addressed by a separate study. For example, the challenges facing health professions education or biomedical research have been and will continue to be the subject of focused study. The goal of this committee was to synthesize across these major issues and develop a broad future vision and direction for the roles of AHCs in the 21st century. The challenges are complex; thus it is inevitable that some issues will remain unaddressed in any single report.

CHAPTER 2

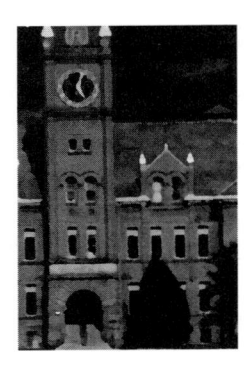

FORCES FOR CHANGE

Although much has been written on the pressures facing AHCs in the current environment, trends already under way will exert enormous pressure on how AHCs will carry out their roles in the future. Profoundly shifting public needs and demands, breathtakingly rapid changes in technology, and unrelenting cost pressures will impose new demands on the entire health care system. AHCs face particularly intense scrutiny and high expectations for meeting these new and evolving demands because of their special roles in education, patient care, and research. As this chapter reveals, these trends necessitate a reexamination of how AHCs carry out those roles to meet the public's health needs.

The first section of the chapter describes the changing environment faced by AHCs and the resulting need for new capabilities. This is followed by a review of the challenges to change within AHCs, which, in combination with the changes described, form the context within which the needed transformation of the AHC roles must occur.

**THE CHANGING ENVIRONMENT AND
THE NEED FOR NEW CAPABILITIES**

Many different forces are driving changes in the environment in which AHCs function. The strongest of these forces can be grouped into three broad categories: (1) changing health care needs, (2) technological advances (including information and biomedical technologies), and (3) continued cost pressures. These major forces necessitate new capabilities—indeed, as many would argue, a paradigm shift—in the health care system of the 21st century.

Changing Health Care Needs

The overall health care needs of people are changing in several ways. One is the shift in disease burden from acute to chronic care. Another is growing recognition of the influence of lifestyle and behavioral choices on health and illness. A third is other demographic shifts that will affect expectations and demands of the health care system.

Chronic Care Needs

During the 20th century, health care delivery focused on the treatment of acute illness, often by solo practitioners in offices and hospitals. In the 21st century, meeting the health needs and expectations of the population will require a focus on chronic rather than acute care. Chronic conditions are now the leading cause of illness, disability, and death in the United States, affecting almost half of the U.S. population and accounting for the majority of health care resources used (Hoffman et al., 1996; Foundation for Accountability and The Robert Wood Johnson Foundation, 2002). Indeed, chronic disease accounts for about 70 percent of all deaths in the United States (Hoffman et al., 1996). The major chronic disease killers are cardiovascular disease, cancer, diabetes, and chronic obstructive pulmonary disease (Centers for Disease Control and Prevention, 2001). Although a greater proportion of the over-65 population has chronic conditions relative to other age groups, the majority of people with chronic conditions are under age 65 (Institute of Medicine, 2001b).

Care for those with chronic conditions is one of the major drivers in the use of health resources. Costs for care of people with chronic disease account for more than 60 percent of the nation's total medical care costs (National Center for Chronic Disease Prevention and Health Promotion, 1999). Compared with people with acute conditions, annual medical costs per person were more than double for people with one chronic condition and almost six times higher for those with two or more such conditions (The Robert Wood Johnson Foundation, 1996). People with chronic conditions also spend more out of their own pockets for health care. In 1996, average out-of-pocket spending for those without a chronic condition was $249, as compared with $1,134 for those with three or more such conditions (Hwang et al., 2001).

People with chronic conditions make different demands on the health care system than those requiring acute care. They use more health care and a wider variety of services, and higher costs are associated with their care (Hoffman et al., 1996; The Robert Wood Johnson Foundation, 1996). They use multiple specialist services and more home health care and nonhospital services, and they face greater need for coordination and communication along the continuum of care. The current health care delivery system is woefully inadequate in meeting these demands (Wagner et al., 2001; Anderson and Knickman, 2001). It has been estimated that fewer than half of patients with hypertension, depression, diabetes, and asthma are receiving appropriate treatment (Wagner et al., 2001).

Lifestyle Influences on Health

Behavioral risk factors, such as smoking, heavy drinking, and obesity, are known risk factors for illness and disease. Significant levels of illness and death are strongly correlated with behavior patterns that could be modified (McGinnis et al., 2002). Obesity is associated with a 36 percent increase in inpatient and outpatient spending (Grumbach, 1999). Cigarette smoking is the leading cause of preventable deaths in the United States. Between 1995 and 1999, smoking caused approximately 440,000 premature deaths, and smoking-related medical expenditures totaled more than $75 billion in 1998 alone (Fellows et al., 2002). Although the impact of behavior on chronic conditions is known, people report not receiving the information they need to manage their illnesses successfully. For example, 40 percent of people with hypertension say they were not advised to limit salt intake or control their weight (Foundation for Accountability and The Robert Wood Johnson Foundation, 2002).

Improving health status will require a better understanding of the determinants of health and illness and of how to educate people about and influence the lifestyle and behavioral choices that affect the prevalence and severity of chronic conditions. Such understanding is needed at the individual patient level, but stronger interventions are needed at the population level as well to achieve broader change.

Other Demographic Shifts

The population of the United States is slowly aging in both absolute and relative terms. About 13 percent of the population is currently over age 65; this proportion is estimated to increase to 20 percent by 2030 (National Center for Health Statistics, 1999). The aging of the baby boom generation in particular is expected to transform many aspects of society, although the effect on the health and welfare system will not be felt substantially until 2030, when the youngest members of that generation reach age 65 (Institute for the Future, 2000).

The aging of the population, as well as a sharp drop in fertility rates during the 1960s and 1970s, will result in slower growth of the labor force in future years (Davis, 2002). It has been estimated that the number of workers per retiree will decline from about 4.75 in 2010 to about 2.75 in 2040 (American Health Care Association, 2002), with implications for funding levels for Social Security and Medicare. The shift in demographics will also result in an increasingly tight labor market that can be expected to exert upward pressure on the wages of health workers, increasing demand to improve productivity in health care (Davis, 2002).

The population is also becoming more diverse. Although 73 percent of the U.S. population is Caucasian non-Hispanic, the Hispanic, Asian, African American, and Native American populations are all growing more rapidly than the population as a whole. By 2010, minority ethnic and racial groups will account for 32 percent of the nation's population (Institute for the Future, 2000). Among those 65 and older, approximately 14 percent are minorities; this proportion is expected to reach 50 percent by 2100 (Wolf, 2001). Hispanics are projected to be as large as all other minority groups combined (Wolf, 2001). The importance of these trends is that disparities in health remain for different population groups. For example, chronic conditions appear to differ in their prevalence among racial groups and low-income and disadvantaged populations (Foundation for Accountability and The Robert Wood Johnson Foundation, 2002; Wolf, 2001).

These general demographic shifts have at least three major implications. First, the growing diversity of the population will result in increased variation in people's expectations of the health care system, creating demands for greater cultural sensitivity and competency in the system's design and from its practitioners. Second, the aging and diversity of the population will have significant implications for the availability, mix, and price of the health care workforce. Finally, the growth of the population covered by Medicare, combined with relatively fewer people paying into the system, is likely to force trade-offs to maintain financing, such as reducing benefits, raising taxes, or allowing larger deficits (Strunk and Ginsburg, 2002).

Technological Advances

As discussed here, the term "technological advances" encompasses a range of technology-based capabilities, including information technology; telecommunications and systems analysis; biotechnology, genomics, proteomics, and structural biology; and imaging and clinical applications. The effects of these advances will be profound, affecting what kind of care is provided to people, when it is provided, where it is provided, and by whom. The result is likely to be a redefinition of what constitutes health and medical care. The impacts of advances in two of these areas—information and communications technology, and biotechnology—are reviewed below.

Information and Communications Technology

Inaccessible or poor-quality information has been identified as one of the health sector's most avoidable shortcomings (Detmer, 2003). Public health agencies are unable to share critical information quickly or pool data for analysis; treatment advances take too long to reach people, while unproven procedures are widely used; variation in practice patterns means that the costs and outcomes of care that people experience depend on where they live rather than scientific evidence; and both patients and clinicians face conflicting and poor-quality information.

Information and communications technologies (discussed here under the rubric of information technology for the sake of brevity) have the power to transform health and medical care. The information technologies expected to have the greatest impact on health care are clinical information and decision support systems, the electronic medical record, and Internet-based health interactions (Institute for the Future, 2000).

Applications of information technology in clinical care can range from simple automation of tasks that improve the speed of transactions to complex knowledge management that includes adaptive clinical decision support systems (Institute of Medicine, 2001b). Information technology can affect clinical decision making by enabling real-time data to be available where clinical decisions are made. Individual patient data can be accessed, as well as comparative data and information about current evidence and best practice. Using information technology, virtual teams in different locations can confer about a patient without ever meeting face to face, a capability with the potential to improve efficiency and continuity of care. Information technology can also improve clinical efficiency by reducing errors and variations in practice. Computer-based physician order-entry systems have been shown to reduce medication errors by more than 50 percent (Doolan and Bates, 2002). Information technology can yield cost savings as well. For example, one estimate suggests that the clinical information system at Vanderbilt University Medical Center enabled $7 million in operating savings in just 1 year by controlling drug costs and improving the flow of information, which made it possible to meet increases in patient volume without adding staff (Morrissey, 2002).

Information technology can also allow people to become more involved in their own care through improved access to information. The Internet is a strong influence in encouraging such involvement (Kassirer, 2000; Kleinke, 2000; Starr, 2000), and the proportion of active users of the Internet among the U.S. population quadrupled between 1995 and 2000

(Starr, 2000). Through the Internet, patients are able to learn more about treatment options and connect with others experiencing the same problem to receive support for self-management or trade information (Fried et al., 2000). The Internet can be especially powerful for people with chronic conditions. It makes continuous monitoring possible by allowing patients and their clinicians to stay in touch on a regular basis without relying on face-to-face visits (Starr, 2000). Telemedicine will be able to expand beyond its historical role of bringing services to rural populations as online consultations, especially with video and data links, become a reality, making care less place dependent (Starr, 2000). Information that may have been inaccessible or could come only from a physician can now be easily accessed and printed by patients anytime, anywhere (Kleinke, 2000; Fried et al., 2000). Access to such resources allows patients to take a greater role in treatment decisions, and may necessitate different approaches when health professionals counsel their patients. Many believe that, despite concerns regarding security, privacy, and malpractice, the Internet is poised to become a major vehicle for health care (Kassirer, 2000).

Information technology is expected to have a significant effect on measurement and surveillance as well. Information technology creates opportunities to analyze large amounts of data and to measure outcomes of care, especially at the population level. The ability to conduct better analyses of clinical performance and cost-effectiveness and to track changes over time can improve significantly. Information technology is also expected to support enhanced surveillance so that disease outbreaks and bioterrorism can be detected quickly, and to create the opportunity to link public health and acute care delivery systems for improved response (Salinksy, 2002; Agency for Healthcare Research and Quality, 2002).

Finally, information technology will have a major effect on overall work design in health care by influencing how the work is conducted, what roles and responsibilities are assumed, and how people work together. For example, information technology is likely to permit functions traditionally performed by physicians to be performed by other clinicians (Christensen et al., 2000; Weed and Weed, 1999). This change will in turn raise fundamental issues regarding how human capital is deployed, influencing projections of the supply, mix, and distribution of needed labor. Past projections have often focused on the supply of physicians or the mix of specialists and generalists (see, for example, reports by the Council of Graduate Medical Education). Few studies have examined the roles of nonphysician clinicians, such as advanced nurse practitioners, nurse midwives, or physician assistants (Cooper et al., 1998; Grumbach and Coffman, 1998). Yet projections of workforce needs based on the assumption that work processes will remain the same will be insufficient for assessing future needs.

Biotechnology

Biotechnology offers great promise for improving health and preventing disease. Biotechnology encompasses the use of cellular and molecular processes to solve problems or develop products (Biotechnology Industry Organization, 2003). In health care, it has been applied in the development of medicines, vaccines, diagnostic tools, and gene therapy. Among the most promising areas are genomics, with its potential to predict disease and improve diagnosis, and proteomics, or understanding of the complete set of proteins that make up a living organism. Knowing the genes and their proteins is one essential component of understanding physiology and explaining disease (Fontanarosa and DeAngelis, 2002). The complexity presented by 35,000 human genes and 100,000 proteins is enormous, but it is believed that the molecular basis of most human diseases will eventually be explained (Pollard, 2002). A related and emerging area is structural biology, which includes the study of biological macromolecules from a structural perspective (National Institutes of Health, 2002). It comprises a number of subdisciplines, such as x-ray diffraction, electron microscopy, computational biology, chemistry, and engineering.

Advances in gene testing could make it possible to identify the potential for the development of a disease and to undertake early interventions to avoid, delay, or moderate symptoms (Myers et al., 2001). Preventive care would take on an entirely different meaning (Samuels, 2001). The ability to intervene early in a disease process, perhaps prior to the emergence of symptoms, would alter the very definition of medicine, health, and preventive care. Applied to pharmaceutical development, pharmacogenomics could make it possible to genetically engineer therapies and individualize the design of a drug to make it safer and more effective (Robertson et al., 2002). Expectations are high that diagnosis, treatment, and prevention will advance rapidly as a result of these advances.

Moreover, biotechnology will converge with information technology to create several new areas for research not possible in the past. Bioengineering, bioinformatics, computational biology, and nanotechnology are among such promising areas for future research.

Clinical imaging is another promising area on the long list of biomedical possibilities. Developments in established fields, such as light and electron microscopy, and in new fields, such as scanning probe and magnetic resonance imaging microscopy, combine advances in hardware and computer algorithms to improve resolution and structural detail at the molecular and cellular levels (Office of Extramural Research, 2002).

In the area of neurological diseases, neuroscientists are applying new understandings in modern genetics and information derived from the sequencing of the human genome to gain insight into the hundreds of disorders that afflict the nervous system, advancing the treatment of spinal cord injury, acute stroke, multiple sclerosis, and Parkinson's disease. Progress in research on the channels, synapses, and circuit structures of the body at the atomic level offer the greatest opportunity for applying methods by which new drugs are targeted for the treatment of epilepsy, pain, movement disorders, and neuromuscular disorders (National Institute of Neurological Disorders and Stroke, 1999). Advances in imaging technology, such as positron emission tomography (PET) and functional magnetic resonance imaging (fMRI), have brought about a revolution in the study of cognition and behavior. As a result, the opportunity now exists to detect early changes in brain function and assist in understanding the mechanisms of such diseases as autism.

The list could go on, but it is clear that these and other scientific advances will produce an explosion of knowledge that is just getting under way today. To derive the benefits of such advances, however, efforts at translating the knowledge gained from research into clinical practice need to be "substantially improved" (Frist, 2002, p. 1723). Clinical trials are important for translating research from the bench to the bedside, but a significant leap beyond clinical trials is required to transform health care practice to reflect the latest advances.

Continued Cost Pressures

Persistent cost pressures threaten all avenues of progress in health care. After a slowdown in the growth of health care expenditures for several years, recent trends suggest a faster rate of growth may be recurring (Ginsburg, 1999). In 2001, health care spending rose a nominal 8.7 percent, well above the average growth rate of 5.7 percent between 1993 and 2000. Adjusting for inflation, this figure represents a real rate of growth of 6.2 percent (Levit et al., 2003). The Centers for Medicare and Medicaid Services projects that health care spending will continue to grow through 2008 at an average annual rate of 6.8 percent, reaching $2.2 trillion or 16 percent of gross domestic product (Blumenthal, 2001).

The growth in spending on health care is being reflected in premium costs for health insurance and increased out-of-pocket spending by patients. Between 2000 and 2001, monthly premiums for employer-sponsored health insurance rose 11 percent, up from an average increase of 8.3 percent in the prior year (Kaiser Family Foundation and Health Research and Educational Trust, 2001). Smaller firms (fewer than 200 workers) saw premium increases of 12.5 percent, compared with 10.2 percent for larger firms. This increase in premiums is the greatest since 1992, and the trend is expected to continue. In 2003, for example, the California Public Employees' Retirement System is facing increases in excess of 20 percent (Consumer Reports, 2002).

Higher expenditures are also reflected in increased cost-sharing requirements for patients. Both deductibles and copayments have risen in all types of health plans provided to employees (Gabel et al., 2001). As health care expenditures rise, employers and payers are indicating their intention to increase consumer cost sharing (Robinson, 2002). Tiered pricing plans are one potential means of putting more decision making into the hands (and pockets) of consumers. The proportion of health plans offering a three-tier design for pharmaceuticals (varying out-of-pocket costs for generic, brand-name, and nonformulary drugs) rose to 80 percent in 2000, up from 36 percent in 1998 (Mays et al., 2001). The same concept is being applied to hospital choice. Some health plans in selected markets are varying consumer out-of-pocket payments for different hospitals that are tiered according to their costs. Consumers who choose to use AHCs, which are typically more expensive than other hospitals, may face higher out-of-pocket spending for that choice (Robinson, 2003; Yegian, 2003).

Growing interest in defined contribution plans may also give consumers a greater role in deciding what coverage and services to buy. In defined contribution plans, an employer or other payer contributes a certain amount to the purchase of health insurance by employees or beneficiaries. Those who wish to purchase a more expensive package must pay the difference in cost out of their own pockets (Blumenthal, 2001). About 24 percent of all small firms and 13 percent of all large firms say they are very or somewhat likely to switch to a defined contribution plan over the next 5 years, compared with 20 percent and 16 percent, respectively, in the prior year (Kaiser Family Foundation and Health Research and Educational Trust, 2001).

The degree to which consumers will accept increases in their out-of-pocket costs is unclear, and at some point a backlash could occur as people are forced to balance their desire and expectation for access to care, including the latest technologies, against the costs of care. Nonetheless, a return to the first-dollar coverage seen in prior years is unlikely. Compared with today's system, the system of the coming decades will likely be more consumer driven as patients take on greater responsibility for the costs of their care and are increasingly armed with information to make decisions about their care.

Although the level and rate of increase in health care spending is a concern in and of itself, the concern widens when its impact on other pressing problems is considered. Persistent increases in expenditures threaten to exacerbate already serious problems of access. About 40 million people in the United States, or 17 percent of the population under age 65, are uninsured (Institute of Medicine, 2001a). The number of people without insurance has increased by about 1 million per year, even during years of economic prosperity (Holahan and Kim, 2000). As employer premiums increase, many observers note the potential for still further increases in the number of uninsured (Strunk et al., 2001). Although access limitations are more severe for people with no insurance, even those with health insurance are concerned about their access to care because of copayments, deductibles, or insufficient coverage. Among five industrialized nations, the United States has the highest percentage of people who report having problems paying medical bills (Schoen et al., 2002). Increased costs make it difficult to maintain equitable access for vulnerable populations to basic as well as specialized services.

Recognized and serious quality problems also make it clear that the resources being devoted to health care are not producing the desired results (Institute of Medicine, 2001b). Standard practices are increasingly being questioned. Arthroscopic surgery for arthritic knees and long-term hormone replacement therapy for women, for example, have recently been found to be ineffective and possibly even harmful for some patients (Moseley et al., 2002; Writing Group for the Women's Health Initiative Investigators, 2002). Assumptions about the management of patients with atrial fibrillation that have been unquestioned for many years have been recently found to be "wanting" (Falk, 2002, p. 1883). Some patients receive services that provide no benefit, while others fail to receive services that could help. For example:

- Preventable medication errors alone were shown to harm approximately 500 patients per year in a large teaching hospital (Chassin et al., 1998).
- Fully 45 percent of diabetics reported that they had not received three recommended annual checks (eye exam, foot exam, and blood pressure) (Davis, 2002).
- Only 50 percent of eligible adults above age 65 receive the recommended yearly influenza vaccine, and only 28 percent receive the indicated pneumococcal vaccine (James, 2001).
- Studies conducted between 1987 and 1997 suggest that about 20 percent of care for chronic conditions was provided without appropriate clinical indications (Becher and Chassin, 2001).

Better ways of delivering care to people are needed so that care is safe, effective, patient-centered, timely, efficient, and equitable (Institute of Medicine, 2001b). Developing better models of care represents one piece of the puzzle in addressing the pressures on the costs of care. One study estimates that quality problems such as overuse, misuse, and waste represent 30 percent of the direct costs of health care, or about $390 billion in 2000, excluding the indirect costs of lost workdays (Midwest Business Group on Health et al., 2002). This estimate is consistent with those of other studies. If the wide variation that exists across the country in the use of medical services were reduced, it has been estimated that Medicare spending could be decreased by about 29 percent (Wennberg et al., 2002). These various studies suggest that cost savings, to some degree, are possible.

Given the pressures that employers, consumers, and other payers are now facing for the costs of care, additional funds are likely to be accompanied by calls for greater accountability and an understanding of the value being derived from current investments and the resource choices being made. Providers that rely on public sources of support are also likely to be affected by efforts to control spending.

Needs and Expectations for the 21st Century

Collectively, the trends described in this chapter are considered by some to represent a paradigm shift. The Institute for the Future (2000) views the paradigm shift in health care as the movement from a biomedical model to a model that employs a broader view of health. The biomedical model is characterized by a focus on the acute care episode, the individual patient and his or her disease, and the goal of curing the disease. In contrast, the broader view of health will focus on managing chronic illness, attending to the needs of populations as well as individuals, and adapting to diseases with no cure.

At the Duke Private Sector Conference of 2000 (Snyderman and Saito, 2000), Snyderman described a paradigm shift from a reactive to a proactive health care model. The reactive model is characterized by a focus on the treatment of disease at the time that a patient presents for treatment, an emphasis on sporadic interventions, physician-directed care based on experience, and care that is cost insensitive. In contrast, the proactive model will involve using an understanding of genetic susceptibility and behavioral risk to predict and prevent disease, taking interactive approaches to care, and emphasizing clinical decision making that is evidence based and cost sensitive.

The Institute of Medicine's (2001b) report *Crossing the Quality Chasm: A New Health System for the 21st Century* describes a paradigm shift from what can be viewed as a provider-centered to a patient-centered system. The former is characterized by a focus on visits, professional autonomy, experience-based decision making, and secrecy. In contrast, the patient-centered system will focus on continuous healing relationships between patients and their care team, cooperation among clinicians, care that is driven by patient needs and values, evidence-based decision making, and transparency.

The Blue Ridge Academic Health Group (1998a) describes a value-driven health system that is characterized by a focus on advancing health, as distinct from delivering medical services. This system has six dimensions:

(1) universal health coverage so that competition can be based on quality and efficiency; (2) management of population health through the allocation of public health resources and collaborations between public health and health care professionals; (3) identification, communication, and management of individual and population health risks before the onset of disease and associated treatment costs; (4) the participation of all health care delivery organizations in a community or region in efforts to advance health, with contributions by AHCs to an improved understanding of population health through their research and education; (5) the measurement of performance by all health care organizations and accountability within the organization and to the community for resource use; and (6) the presence of a robust information technology infrastructure to manage knowledge for delivery organizations, professionals, and patients, and to enable data collection and analysis, as well as access to available evidence.

Some believe the current health system is overly focused on meeting the needs of a relatively small population of very sick patients. Because of this, it is vulnerable to disruption by technologies and other innovations that can offer cheaper, simpler, and more convenient means of care that will meet the relatively straightforward needs of the majority of the population (Christensen et al., 2000).

Whether or not history will reveal this era as a paradigm shift, there is no question that the factors described in this chapter will have a significant impact. The combined effects of these factors will be especially powerful and can be expected to produce at least three broad trends for health care.

First, patients will exert more direction and control over their care. Greater patient involvement in care associated with the management of chronic illness, combined with increased responsibility for the costs of care and greater access to information, will result in patients wanting and having greater direction over their care. Evidence for this trend can already be seen. Information about health care is one of the most common objects of searches on the Internet. People are seeking information on complementary and alternative medicine in record numbers, suggesting an openness and willingness to pursue alternative forms of therapy outside the mainstream health system (National Center for Complementary and Alternative Medicine, 2001). Over-the-counter home testing products are expanding rapidly into many different uses, presenting the opportunity for people to test themselves at home for conditions that may previously have required an office visit and a prescription, and permitting patients to become their own diagnosticians.

Second, there will be greater interest in a more lifelong, integrative view of medicine and health. Managing chronic illness over an extended period of time requires more than just good medical care; it also requires an involved and educated patient, behavioral and lifestyle changes, and good coordination between medical care and other services (often community-based) that can support health maintenance. Increasing costs of care and greater individual responsibility for those costs should foster greater interest in approaches for staying healthy among both patients and payers. A more integrated view will also be supported by interest in maximizing the benefits of scientific advances. Biomedical advances that offer opportunities for early intervention and prevention of disease will fail to provide their maximum benefit if they are not accessed until a patient exhibits symptoms and presents for treatment. Needs related to managing illness, controlling costs, and maximizing scientific advances will increase interest in both the medical and nonmedical determinants of health and illness.

Third, there will be greater pressure to measure and understand value in health care. Increased patient decision making, especially in the face of rising costs, along with information technology that can support improved analysis and measurement, will result in increased demand to understand what does and does not work in health care. Greater pressure will be placed on applying what we know works and discontinuing what we know does not work. Improving value will require making care safer and reducing errors in all settings. As science continues to advance, there will be increased calls for understanding how to apply the resulting discoveries effectively. Having the scientific potential to reduce illness and improve health, as well as the information technology and tools to understand and apply the advances achieved, will make patients, payers, and policy makers impatient for the enhanced care thus enabled.

CHALLENGES TO CHANGE WITHIN AHCS

The changes described above affect all health care organizations and professionals. In addition, however, AHCs face a number of unique challenges that also exert pressure for change.

AHCs have traditionally funded their activities through a complex system of cross-subsidies that is being disrupted (Iglehart, 1994). About 90 percent of total AHC revenues is derived from clinical care; these revenues are used to cross-subsidize activities in research and education (The Commonwealth Fund Task Force on Academic Health Centers, 1997b). Until the early 1990s, AHCs had a bounty of resources and were able to operate with relatively few concerns for efficiency (Beller, 2000; Galvin, 2002). In the mid- to late 1990s, however, the situation appeared to change, and AHCs began to experience increased financial pressures as rising costs of care constrained payments from both public and private payers. These pressures affected AHCs in particular, whose average costs are approximately 25 to 30 percent higher than those of other hospitals (Blumenthal and Meyer, 1996; Kassirer, 1994). Payment constraints increased pressure on faculty to generate clinical revenues, creating concerns that attention is being diverted from education and research (Beller, 2000; Blumenthal and Meyer, 1996; DeAngelis, 2000).

AHCs also face challenges to the financial support they receive for each of their roles. Although AHCs have raised questions about the adequacy of funding for graduate medical education, some observers have questioned whether such subsidy should be provided at all (Newhouse and Wilensky, 2001; Gbadebo and Reinhardt, 2001). In terms of research funding, AHCs have expressed concerns about their ability to continue to sustain research activities that are not supported with external funds, including activities associated with conducting the preliminary work required to develop new ideas and seek grants, some capital expenses, and the institutional contribution required by some funders (such as NIH), which are estimated to represent 15 to 20 percent of a project's total expenses (The Commonwealth Fund Task Force on Academic Health Centers, 1999; Weissman, et al., 1999). AHCs have been major beneficiaries of the increases in federal support for health-related research, but it is not clear that historical rates of increase can be sustained into the future, and this situation could potentially affect the funding stream available to support AHC research activities (Korn, 2002).

One recent report notes that between 1994 and 2000, the financial resources available to AHCs to support their core roles in education, research, and patient care diminished (Dobson et al., 2002). The aggregate total and operating margins of AHC hospitals were lower in 2000 than in any year since 1994, a decline attributed to decreases in payments from private providers and, especially for public AHCs, increases in uncompensated care. Analyses by the Medicare Payment Advisory Commission found that the decline in total hospital margins may have halted in 2002, although these analyses did not separate out the experience of AHC hospitals (Medicare Payment Advisory Commission, 2003). Moreover, these analyses examined the financial status of the hospital only. The complexity of the AHCs makes it difficult to get a clear sense of their overall financial status, since the experience of that of the hospital may not be representative of the whole AHC. For example, the Hospital of the University of Pennsylvania reported a 1999 operating margin of −11 percent, while the operating margin of its obligated group (the affiliates that share long-term debt) was 9 percent (Kane, 2001).

Not all the challenges facing AHCs are financial, however. From an organizational perspective, AHCs tend to be large, complex entities that are loosely affiliated arrangements (see Chapter 1). As they face today's competitive marketplace and a rapidly changing delivery system, their size and organizational complexity make decision making slow and often cumbersome (Galvin, 2002). This is especially true for decisions that need to be made at the level of the overall AHC enterprise (as opposed to the departmental level) (Iglehart, 1995). The size and complexity of AHCs also present an obstacle to partnering with other organizations (Galvin, 2002).

AHCs have to respond to an exceptionally diverse number of constituencies. To carry out their many activities, they must satisfy patients, purchasers, faculty, employees, students, the broader research community, funders, accrediting agencies, state and federal policy makers, alumni, local communities, community-based facilities and providers, and other partners. They operate with one foot in the university and one foot in the competitive marketplace. They are providers of last resort for the uninsured who need care and have nowhere else to turn. They are also providers of last resort for the seriously ill who need the most sophisticated care and have exhausted all other possibilities.

The ability of AHCs to respond to the forces for change influences the capabilities of the rest of the health system. If AHCs do not adapt their activities in education and research to meet changing needs and demands, it will be difficult for the broader health care system to have the trained professionals and knowledge needed to deliver care effectively. Thus, the whole health care system is influenced by the pace at which AHCs are able to adapt their roles to a changing set of demands and expectations placed on the nation's health care system. Certainly, the overall health system is affected by other factors in addition to the activities of AHCs, but the roles performed by AHCs are a major influence in building the health system's overall capacity to adapt to the changes that will affect health care in the coming decades.

Despite the variation in AHCs, this committee believes there is sufficient commonality among them that a set of expectations can be defined for each of their roles. This does not mean that all AHCs will do the same thing or carry out activities in the same way. AHCs will still choose varying paths to balance their different roles in accordance with local needs and resource availability. But it is indeed possible and reasonable to clarify expectations for the AHC roles, and even advisable given the public dollars that support the AHCs' work.

CHAPTER 3

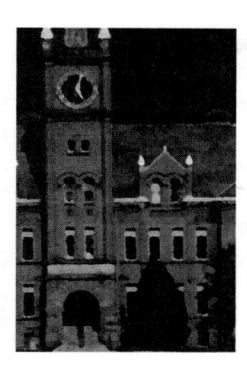

THE ACADEMIC HEALTH CENTER AS A REFORMER: THE EDUCATION ROLE

The forces described in Chapter 2 demand a change in the approaches and attributes of clinical education in the 21st century. Demographic changes, technological and scientific advances, and continued cost pressures necessitate a reexamination of how health professionals are prepared for practice. The committee finds the following:

- AHCs have played a major role in the education of health professionals, successfully teaching the latest procedures and interventions for relieving the symptoms and suffering of sick patients. They have emphasized in particular the education of physicians at the undergraduate and graduate levels, relying on the hospital's inpatient and outpatient settings as primary training sites.
- The AHC role in education for the 21st century will require more than the direct training of health professionals. AHCs will be expected to demonstrate leadership in the design and development of educational approaches for health professionals throughout the continuum of education. Doing so will require much more than curricular reform, requiring consideration of how the clinical settings in which students are trained reinforces the attributes desired of health professionals in the 21st century.
- All teaching environments will need to provide a sound base of knowledge that includes not only the emerging sciences, such as genomics, but also the social, behavioral, and other sciences that are important to

improving health. Providing a broad-based scientific and humanistic foundation will require that all teaching environments reexamine the content, methods, and approaches used at all levels of clinical education, including undergraduate, graduate, and continuing education.

- As part of their education role, AHCs need to work with educators and other resources within their parent universities to develop the evidence base for clinical education so that the approaches used will be based on sound educational principles that improve understanding of the quality of clinical education.

As university-affiliated, academic organizations, AHCs need to take a leadership role in meeting these challenges. The first section of this chapter examines the need for new approaches to clinical education to provide the new skills required for the health care workforce of the future. This is followed by a discussion of the factors that affect the ability of AHCs to reform clinical education. The final section describes some implications for the future.

NEED FOR NEW APPROACHES TO PROVIDE NEW SKILLS

As noted above, the trends and developments described in Chapter 2 will create a different set of expectations for practice and require different types of skills from health professionals. Shifting patient needs, the evolving science of medicine, and changes in the organization and financing of care will all affect how health professionals should be prepared for practice. Health professionals trained today can be expected to reach their peak of practice around 2040, a health environment that is sure to be very different from that of today.

There is no question that additional skills will be required. For example, the greater understanding of the mechanisms of disease that will be possible with genetic and other scientific advances will improve diagnosis and treatment, but also make them more complex. Analysis of disease at the molecular level will move diagnosis to that level as well (Pollard, 2002). Clinicians will require skills in differentiating genetic, other, and combined sources of illness. This requirement will alter the skills needed for diagnosis; moreover, treatments will have to be individualized to accommodate expected responses to treatment given a patient's genetic profile. These skills will not be demanded only of specialists; genetics will also redefine how primary care and preventive medicine are practiced. Changes in the organization and financing of care will require that health professionals demonstrate safe, efficient, and effective practice styles. Changing patient needs will necessitate increased emphasis on skills required to manage chronic conditions, including, for example, understanding the course of illness and the patient's experience outside the hospital, with a focus on prevention, behavioral change, and maximizing of functioning.

The education of health professionals for future practice involves more than identifying needed skills, however. In health care, students learn through a combination of classroom experience and supervised clinical practice. In fact, the bulk of health professions training is in the latter venue. Although the situation is changing, the first 2 years of medical school are focused most heavily on learning the basic sciences in a classroom setting. The last 2 years consist of clinical rotations, followed by at least 3 years of residency, also in a clinical setting. Therefore, the clinical experience represents about 70 percent of medical training. In nursing, it is estimated that about 50 percent of training for baccalaureate-prepared registered nurses is in clinical settings, and the proportion increases with advanced training (Helen Bednash, personal communication, Jan. 10, 2003). The clinical learning environment, sometimes referred to as the informal curriculum, communicates values, culture, personal development, priorities, and the language of the field to students (Accreditation Council for Graduate Medical Education, 2002). It influences their relationships with each other and with patients.

To prepare health professionals for practice in the coming decades, therefore, the clinical experience must be addressed. It is not enough to say what should be taught to students; it is also necessary to consider the context in which it is taught and the approaches used, and how knowledge, skills, and attitudes are both acquired and taught. A focus on skills considers the competencies required of students at the conclusion of a training program, while a focus on the clinical experience considers the "competencies" or capabilities of the training program itself, focusing on what is conveyed, and how, during the clinical experience.

As noted in Chapter 2, the changing environment of health care will have at least three consequences that can be expected to affect the education of health professionals. First, patients will exert more influence over their care decisions, both because they will bear the costs of care and because they will be faced with making more choices as technology expands treatment options. Second, there will be increased calls to measure and manage care as costs increase in the face of concerns about quality and access and as information technology makes it more feasible to do so. Third, improving health will require a broader view in which the discoveries of science and the new biology combine with those of the social and behavioral sciences to affect the determinants of health and illness.

Given these trends and directions, the committee identifies three approaches that will need to be considered by all training programs in the coming decades: interdisciplinary approaches that ensure a broader view of health, tools and methods for managing information, and training in nonhospital settings. Each is briefly discussed below. It should be noted that although some progress is being made toward implementing these approaches, current educational programs are focused at the departmental and discipline-specific levels; as a result, varied levels of commitment and resources are devoted to such approaches, even within a single AHC. Significant advances in health professions education will require a clear commitment and adequate resources across the entire AHC.

Interdisciplinary Approaches and a Broader View of Health

Interdisciplinary education occurs when "faculty learn, work and teach together" (Gelmon, 1996, p. 218) to prepare students to work as a team driven by the health needs of patients and the goal of providing the services necessary to improve health to the extent possible (Bulger, 2000; Gelmon, 1996). Interdisciplinary education involves more than simply defining the roles of various clinicians (Osterweis, 2001). Health professionals that are well prepared for practice in the 21st century will collaborate across departments and disciplines, and even settings of care, to meet patients' needs.

The term "interdisciplinary" as used here refers to the involvement of different disciplines, such as medicine, nursing, and pharmacy; the term is not used to denote different specialties within a single discipline, such as internal medicine, cardiology, and endocrinology. The notion of interdisciplinary education will assume increasing significance in the future. For example, the needs of people with chronic conditions (who, as noted in Chapter 2, represent a growing proportion of the population) cannot be met by any single health professional. Similarly, applying the latest biomedical advances will increasingly require the expertise of specialized health professionals, such as genetic counselors. Additionally, if patients are expected to be more accountable for maintaining their health and to assume responsibility for self-care in managing chronic conditions, they also need to be recognized as a key member of the health care team. Yet team interactions in practice often fall short of expectations, in part as a result of current approaches in clinical education that emphasize hierarchy, individual decision making, and the organization of work around professional roles rather than patient needs (Institute of Medicine, 2001b). Indeed, the implementation of more interdisciplinary educational approaches will require a level of cooperation that has rarely been demonstrated. As one observer notes, interdisciplinary training is a "goal often espoused but rarely pursued" (LeRoy, 1994, p.337).

As suggested above, clinical education in the 21st century will also need to take a broader view of medicine and health, with greater emphasis on understanding the social, behavioral, cultural, and environmental factors that influence health and disease in addition to understanding the biological basis of disease (LeRoy, 1994; Josiah Macy, Jr. Foundation, 1999; Young and Coffman, 1998). Developing this understanding will in turn require that biomedical science be better integrated with a patient- and population-based approach that addresses the determinants of disease and health, and places greater emphasis on prevention (LeRoy, 1994) and the identification of risk factors and how to mitigate them.

The focus on the biomedical basis of disease that characterizes the current model for clinical education assumes that ill health is fully explained by disease, so that the core of medical science is the diagnosis and treatment of disease (Cassell, 1999). American medicine, however, is being asked to move beyond this model to address issues related to population health, resource allocation, new means for caring for chronic disease, and the management of health information, all areas in which physicians have traditionally not been trained (Schneider and Eisenberg, 1998). Medical schools in particular are believed to produce physicians well equipped to deal with specific organ systems or pathologies, but ill equipped to deal with the behavioral causes of chronic diseases or the social context of illness (Cantor et al., 1993). According to one survey of young physicians, fewer than half reported receiving excellent or good preparation in coordinating patient care with community services, providing cost-effective care, or managing the needs of the frail elderly (Cantor et al., 1993). Nursing tends to be more oriented toward health promotion and disease prevention. Advanced-practice nurses in particular are focused on establishing knowledge partnerships with their patients, educating them about their conditions, and engaging them in illness prevention and health promotion (Mundinger, 2002).

There are a number of barriers to conducting interdisciplinary education, including turf battles, academic credit, recognition of faculty, and scheduling (Gelmon, 1996; Osterweis, 2001). Each college, even each department, guards its own curriculum, and bringing different students together can be viewed as virtually impossible (Kaufman, 1999). The differing academic schedules of schools can also create a significant obstacle (Osterweis, 2001). Although 60 AHCs have identified an individual with responsibility for interdisciplinary education, only about a dozen have established significant activities in this area; most of the latter are public and community-based, have multiple health professional schools, and fall under the broad jurisdiction of an AHC leader (Osterweis, 2001).

Another potential barrier is that faculty may have neither the skills nor the incentives to pursue interdisciplinary approaches to education. Faculty who themselves have not been trained through interdisciplinary approaches may find it difficult to teach that way and be unable to undertake the educational innovations required to implement such approaches. Moreover, interdisciplinary education is not as strongly rewarded as the efforts of independent scientists working in their laboratories. A concern is that students are not being taught explicitly to work in interdisciplinary teams, but implicitly through the work environment (Conway-Welch, 2002; Larson, 2001), which often has not fostered the types of positive, constructive interactions desired across the disciplines. Strengthening efforts to improve the health of patients and populations will necessitate the development of new educational models.

Conducting rounds with students in multiple disciplines is one approach used for encouraging interdisciplinary interactions, but this approach becomes more difficult to implement as hospital stays shorten. It may be relatively easy to design interdisciplinary education for the classroom, but doing so becomes more difficult in a clinical setting, especially as training diversifies into nonhospital clinical sites. Interdisciplinary approaches also become more difficult to implement when attempted across settings of care. For example, there may be opportunities to foster interdisciplinary training between doctors and nurses in a hospital, but it is less clear how to bring public health into the training model. Some have recommended that public health training be incorporated into medical and nursing schools and that schools of medicine and nursing partner with schools of public health to develop interdisciplinary and joint programs (Institute of Medicine, 2003c). Examples of improved public health training for medical students can be found at Duke University, the University of California at San Francisco, and the University of Southern California (Institute of Medicine, 2003c).

Information Management

Health professionals will need to be prepared to manage information so they can deal with a constantly growing evidence base, serve as an information resource, support decision making by patients, and measure care so they can manage it effectively.

Technological and biomedical advances are expanding the evidence base for health and medical care exponentially. The number of clinical trials published in the literature grew from approximately 1,000 in 1966 to more than 10,000 in 1996, with half that growth experienced in more recent years (Chassin, 1998). This growth in information, which will only intensify in the future, will challenge traditional approaches to educating health professionals. Some have even suggested that the traditional emphasis on a core of knowledge is questionable in light of the expansiveness and dynamic nature of the science base (Weed and Weed, 1999). Rather than the traditional approach based on teaching facts, students should be prepared for the types of problem solving they will face in practice (Weed, 1981).

Health professionals will have to know how to obtain and manage new knowledge as it continually emerges. The concept of evidence-based practice is that a clinical problem is defined, and published evidence is obtained, appraised, synthesized, and applied to the problem (Welch and Lurie, 2000). However, there are virtually an unlimited number of clinical strategies, and resources for evaluation are limited. Educators need to teach the evidence where it is certain, and students need to learn to how to obtain and apply evidence as it develops, as well as how to make clinical decisions when the evidence is absent or weak (Welch and Lurie, 2000).

The increasing complexity of disease and expanding treatment options will require that health professionals be able to serve as an information resource for their patients. Health professionals will need to bridge the gap between the evidence base and patient knowledge, evaluating the evidence and turning it into information that can be explained to patients so their preferences can be expressed. They will need to synthesize, explain, and interpret information to support patient decisions and self-management. In some cases, the health professional's primary role may be serving as an information consultant and resource to guide and support decision making by more informed patients, rather than performing a clinical intervention. There is some evidence that patients whose informational needs are not adequately met are likely to make more visits and use more resources in their care (Mundinger, 2002). Indeed, some have suggested that this information role is one of the most important therapies provided to patients, with health professionals serving as coach and adviser to support patients' increased direction over their care (Schneider, 2002). This role should be incorporated into the education of all health professionals, but also reinforced through interdisciplinary training that recognizes the varying contributions different team members can make to a patient's care.

The increasing costs of care and concerns about the quality of care will result in growing demands to measure and manage care. The management of information must include a focus on measuring care so it can be continuously improved. Research, patient care, and therefore health professions education will become increasingly reliant on evaluative disciplines, such as clinical epidemiology, informatics, health services research, outcomes analysis, and value management (Detmer, 1997; Wennberg, 2002).

Managing information to the extent that will also be required in the future cannot be done without more-advanced information systems to acquire and manage the level of information that will be needed for practice. Part of delivering state-of-the-art care in the future will be the use of clinical and other information systems. Students will need to be prepared to use information technology as a more central component of health care. Clinical education programs that fail to incorporate state-of-the-art information systems into their training will be unable to prepare students for practice today, let alone tomorrow.

Nonhospital Training Experiences

To prepare health professionals to deliver care in the 21st century, education should correspond to care delivery. The majority of care is delivered to patients in noninpatient and nonhospital settings. Nearly a billion ambulatory visits were made in 1999, compared with 32 million hospitalizations (Eberhardt, 2001). Ambulatory care as discussed here refers not only to hospital outpatient departments, but also to offices, community health centers, managed care organizations, public health departments, long-term care facilities, and even patients' homes. Any location where care is delivered should be considered a potential training site.

The predominant model of education today, especially for physicians, consists of training in the inpatient setting, delivering tertiary care. The advantage of hospital-based training is that students can learn from the most challenging and difficult cases. Hospitals that see a larger volume of similar patients (e.g., cardiology or cancer patients) are also more likely to demonstrate higher-quality care in that field, which is desirable to teach (Institute of Medicine, 2001b). In addition, seeing patients who are admitted for ambulatory-sensitive conditions or for certain chronic conditions should give students an opportunity to learn what factors contributed to the condition so they can not only treat the symptoms but also consider how patients might be able to avoid such hospitalizations in the future. It is easier to conduct education in the inpatient setting because the acute problems seen are more readily specified, and therefore, the educational content is easier to define (Showstack, 1999). Finally, inpatient settings offer a cluster of faculty, other students, and an infrastructure to oversee the educational process.

The inpatient model for clinical education will be increasingly ineffective in the coming decades, however. The rate of hospital admissions has been declining; lengths of stay are becoming shorter; many diagnostic problems are being handled outside the hospital; patients in hospitals have the most complex conditions and therefore present a relatively narrow spectrum of diseases; and the sicker patients admitted require increasingly technical care (Kassirer, 1996; Goroll et al., 2001). These trends give the learner less time to establish a relationship with the patient and to understand the multiple medical, social, psychological, and other factors that affect not only the course of disease, but also the individual's health and well-being. A short hospital stay provides a poor learning opportunity to understand the influence of behavioral and social factors on health or to foster shared decision making (Ewan, 1985). Furthermore, most patients admitted electively to the hospital have been worked up prior to admission, so they arrive not only with a chief complaint, but also with the results of diagnostic and laboratory tests, and sometimes, a diagnosis. The intellectual challenge to the learner is incomplete, and the learning opportunity is affected.

Training in the inpatient setting, therefore, does not sufficiently prepare health professionals for practice or provide adequate exposure to alternative settings of care. A survey of young physicians revealed that more than half believed there was too little training in physician offices, organized care settings (e.g., health maintenance organizations), or long-term care facilities (Cantor et al., 1993). People with chronic illness that is managed effectively may often avoid hospitalization for the condition altogether. Even more care can be expected to move out of the inpatient setting as biomedical advances affect when an illness is identified and how it is treated. Finally, in the marketplace, there is a trend toward the provision of nonspecialized care in community hospitals and other settings; specialty care is becoming more concentrated in AHCs (The Commonwealth Fund Task Force on Academic Health Centers, 2000). As AHCs become relatively more focused on specialty care and caring for patients with specialized needs, they become less able to prepare health professionals for everyday practice. It has been estimated that, on average each month, less than 1 person in 1,000 is admitted to an AHC (Green et al., 2001).

There has been some progress in increasing the amount of training provided in ambulatory settings; however, the majority of ambulatory training remains within hospitals, and only a small proportion takes place in nonhospital settings. Primary care physicians can be expected to practice predominantly in nonhospital settings, and they undergo about two-thirds of their training in ambulatory settings; however, only about one-quarter of their training is provided in community settings and about one-tenth is in managed care settings (Brotherton et al., 2000). Among non–primary care residents, just over one-third of training is in ambulatory settings, but only about 6 percent is in community settings and about 6 percent in managed care settings (Brotherton et al., 2000). Furthermore, the proportion of training time in nonhospital ambulatory settings (community and managed care settings) showed a decline between 1997 and 1999—a trend in the wrong direction.

Among undergraduate medical education programs, teaching in outpatient settings in required clinical clerkships occupied one-third or more of the time in primary care program areas compared with one-quarter or less in non–primary care program areas (Barzansky and Etzel, 2001). On the other hand, between 1984 and 1994, the percentage of all medical students who participated in one or more clerkships increased from just under half to almost three-quarters, and the average number of weeks in ambulatory settings increased as well (The Commonwealth Fund Task Force on Academic Health Centers, 2002).

Baccalaureate nursing programs are also offering more opportunities for clinical training in noninstitutional community settings, including visiting nurse agencies, home care, schools, and hospices (National Advisory

Council on Nurse Education and Practice, 1996). To a lesser extent, training is also provided in such settings as nursing centers, senior citizen centers, and homeless shelters.

Shifting training to ambulatory settings involves more than simply moving or adding training slots. Ambulatory settings will not provide a good learning environment without additional preparation. As a learning environment, they can be unpredictable in terms of the types of patients seen, limited in terms of continuity of care, and variable across sites (Irby, 1995). Short patient visits can make it difficult to provide the observation and feedback needed for teaching (Bowen and Irby, 2002). There is also concern that students in ambulatory settings may lose the conferences, faculty, and general educational surroundings offered by the institutional environment (Kassirer, 1996). Indeed, students rate the quality of their instruction in ambulatory settings lower than that in inpatient settings (The Commonwealth Fund Task Force on Academic Health Centers, 2002).

FACTORS THAT AFFECT THE ABILITY OF AHCS TO REFORM EDUCATION

The preceding discussion is not intended to imply that clinical curricula have been static over time. Indeed, there are many examples of efforts aimed at accomplishing the very types of changes outlined above (Association of American Medical Colleges and the Milbank Memorial Fund, 2000; The Commonwealth Fund Task Force on Academic Health Centers, 2002). The Association of Academic Medical Centers recently launched the Institute for Improvement in Medical Education to examine ways to improve medical education curricula, reform the clinical education of medical students and residents, enhance public health education in medical schools, promote professionalism during medical education, engage in international medical education activities, and better meet the need for continued professional development of physicians once they enter practice (Association of American Medical Colleges, 2003a). And more than half of medical schools (58 percent) reported having a major curriculum review or change under way in 2001 (Barzansky and Etzel, 2001).

Many examples of changes in health professions education can be found at individual AHCs. In one example described at the committee's January 2002 workshop, Hundert (2002) described reforms in the medical education curriculum at the University of Rochester[1] through which the clinical and basic sciences are interwoven throughout the 4-year curriculum. He highlighted a course called Mastering Medical Information that is taught in

---

[1]Dr. Hundert has since joined Case Western Reserve University.

the first 4 weeks and last 2 weeks of the first year, in which students learn how to access and navigate through information, gaining skills in data analysis, biostatistics, and epidemiology. Another unique element of the curriculum is a 1-month clerkship in the fourth year called Community Health Improvement. Several years ago, the University of Rochester added a fourth mission to its portfolio—to make Rochester, New York, "the healthiest city in America." The content of the clerkship is determined by the health department's assessment of local health needs, and varies from providing the pneumococcal vaccine in nursing homes to working with teenagers to get them to quit smoking. The academic content of the clerkship is focused on public health and epidemiology.

The Undergraduate Medical Education for the 21st Century (UME-21) program was a 5-year national demonstration project funded in October 1997 by the Health Resources and Services Administration and administered by the American Association of Colleges of Osteopathic Medicine (2003). Eighteen schools were funded to initiate curricular innovations in undergraduate medical education aimed at supporting graduates in practicing high-quality, population-based, cost-effective medicine while maintaining a commitment to care of the individual.[2] The areas addressed in the reforms included health systems finance and organization; the practice of evidenced based medicine, with emphasis on population health; health care ethics; patient–provider relationships and communication skills; leadership and interdisciplinary teamwork; quality measurement and improvement; systems-based care; medical informatics; and wellness and disease prevention.

At the graduate level, the Accreditation Council for Graduate Medical Education (ACGME) has led a major undertaking to move its accreditation processes toward assessment of competencies or outcomes of the education process (Batalden et al., 2002). Six areas of competency are identified: patient care, medical knowledge, practice-based learning and improvement, professionalism, interpersonal skills and communication, and systems-based practice. These six areas will be used to guide residency program directors in curricular development and residency program requirements as defined by the residency review committees. The American Board of Medical Spe-

---

[2]The medical schools involved are Dartmouth, University of California at San Francisco, University of Miami, University of Nebraska, University of Pennsylvania, University of Pittsburgh, University of Wisconsin, Wayne State University, Case Western Reserve, Eastern Virginia University, Jefferson Medical College of Thomas Jefferson University, Medical College of Pennsylvania—Hahnemann, University of Connecticut, University of Kentucky, University of Massachusetts, University of Minnesota, University of New Mexico, and University of North Carolina at Chapel Hill.

cialties (ABMS), the organization for certifying boards of practicing physicians, has accepted these same competencies, thus offering the potential for coordination and reinforcement of skills at the levels of graduate and continuing education.

Nursing educators also have recognized the need for reform in nursing education. The National Advisory Council on Nurse Education and Practice (1996) has recognized the changing nature and responsibilities of registered nurses. Registered nurses will be asked to manage care along a continuum, work in interdisciplinary teams, integrate clinical knowledge with knowledge of community resources, adapt to changing technologies, demonstrate an ability to communicate, and analyze data. Also recognized is the need to prepare the registered nurse workforce more adequately in the use of nursing informatics to support clinical decision making, consumer education, and interactions with other providers (National Advisory Council on Nurse Education and Practice, 1997).

Specific programs to support change have also been undertaken. For example, the American Association of Colleges of Nursing (2002a) has undertaken a major initiative to support gerontology curriculum development, with support from The John A. Hartford Foundation of New York. Objectives include redesign of existing gerontology curriculum, faculty development, design of innovative clinical experiences, and development of new leaders in geriatric practice. The grant will assist nursing schools in adapting their gerontology curriculum and clinical experiences at both the graduate and undergraduate levels. The expectation is that newly identified competencies will be incorporated into advanced-practice nursing programs and will lead to the development of models of excellence for adoption by the broader nursing education community.

The progress made to date reflects the determination of those directing educational programs, who face a number of obstacles in trying to move clinical education forward. Even when AHCs agree with the goals described in this report, a number of factors affect their ability to implement educational reform. The first of these relates to the accreditation and oversight of education programs. Program requirements should support movement toward the attributes desired for clinical education in the 21st century. The second factor relates to faculty development and organization. If students are to have different educational experiences, faculty must be prepared to impart those experiences. The third factor relates to the weak evidence base for clinical education, which makes it difficult to know which changes will have a positive effect on student preparation for practice. The fourth factor relates to financing. Methods of financing for all AHC roles are discussed in Chapter 6, but here we consider the effect of financing on the design of educational programs.

Oversight of Education Programs

It is estimated that more than 50 groups are involved in the oversight of undergraduate and graduate training programs in the health professions (Gelmon et al., 1999). Some of these groups are identified in Box 3-1. The list intentionally includes the accrediting group for programs in health administration. Although the focus of this chapter is on clinical education, the challenges described also face administrators in terms of both their own education and their support for reform efforts in clinical education. Furthermore, clinicians ought to have knowledge of administrative issues, so it is important to consider programs in health administration when looking at coordination across disciplines.

Continuing education requirements are overseen by yet other groups. Accreditation of continuing medical education programs is offered by the Accreditation Council for Continuing Medical Education. The American Osteopathic Association has a separate council for continuing education. The American Nurses Credentialing Center of the American Nurses Association administers the association's credentialing programs, providing both accreditation of continuing education programs and certification for specialty nursing practice. Unlike undergraduate and graduate training, which have clearly defined requirements, requirements for continuing education vary within disciplines. Some physician specialty boards require continuing medical education hours to maintain specialty certification, whereas other have no such requirement (Federation of State Medical Boards, 2002).

The proliferation of oversight groups has serious implications for reforming the education of health professionals. There has been a tendency toward expansion in recent years as more specialties have been recognized, a phenomenon that tends to increase subspecialties (as they seek recognition) and extends the length and cost of training (LeRoy, 1994). However, the approaches proposed in this report are not discipline specific, but apply to everyone. As a result, it may be necessary to ask 50-plus groups to amend their standards. For example, achieving a goal such as interdisciplinary education would require not only that each group make changes, but also that the groups work together in making those changes. That is likely to be a time-consuming process, and it is not clear that there is a mechanism for the purpose.

Coordination across the continuum of education is also poor. Coordination of oversight of education has been called fragmented and duplicative (Gelmon, 1996). Responsibilities for undergraduate, graduate, and continuing education reside for the most part in separate organizations (Enarson and Burg, 1992). As a result, accreditation divorces residency training programs from professional schools (Hanft, 1988). Feedback loops between the levels of education could improve all. For example, if one of

> **BOX 3-1**
> **A Sample of Accrediting Organizations for**
> **Health Professions Education**
>
> Oversight of health professions training occurs through a combination of public and private regulatory activities. A variety of private agencies accredit the education *programs* for undergraduate, graduate, and continuing education. Accredited programs are eligible to receive public funds to support their activities. *Individuals* who complete such programs are then eligible to receive a license to practice from a state, or after graduate training and thereafter, to sit for certification or recertification. These processes are interrelated educationally in that education programs are expected to prepare health professionals to pass licensure exams, and licensure exams are intended to reflect expectations for practice as defined in the scope-of-practice laws (Safriet, 1994). In general, the purposes of these functions are to ensure minimum levels of quality and to protect consumers through assurance of compliance with established standards of quality. It is also hoped that these processes offer the programs and individuals being evaluated an opportunity for self-evaluation and improvement (Gelmon et al., 1999).
>
> The U.S. Department of Education "recognizes" private organizations that carry out education accreditation. In the case of nurse education, the U.S. Department of Education may recognize a state agency to accredit programs. On behalf of the U.S. Department of Education, accreditation agencies may also be recognized by the Council on Higher Education Accreditation (see www.ed.gov/offices/OPE/accreditation). Accreditation is applied to entire institutions and/or individual programs, departments, or schools of a larger institution.
>
> *Undergraduate allopathic medical education:* Accreditation of allopathic medical schools is overseen by the Liaison Committee on Medical Education (LCME). The majority of its membership is from the American Medical Association and Association of American Medical Colleges, but students and the public are represented as well. Substantive changes in LCME's standards must be approved by the Council of Medical Education of the American Medical Association and the Executive Council of the Association of American Medical Colleges (see www.lcme.org).
>
> *Graduate allopathic medical education:* Accreditation of graduate medical education is overseen by the Accreditation Council for Graduate Medical Education (ACGME) for allopathic education, an umbrella organization with membership from five organizations: the American Board of Medical Specialties, the American Hospital Association, the American Medical Association, the Association of American Medical Colleges, and the Council of Medical Specialty Societies. ACGME accredits residency programs through its residency review committees. There is a residency review committee for each specialty board that sets the standards and guidelines by which a residency program will receive accreditation (see www.acgme.org).

Osteopathic undergraduate and graduate medical education: The American Osteopathic Association (AOA) is the accrediting agency for osteopathic medicine. The AOA Bureau of Professional Coordination coordinates accreditation across the continuum of education through several councils. The Council on Predoctoral Education focuses on undergraduate medical education. The Council on Postdoctoral Training focuses on internships, residencies, preceptorships, and other postgraduate medical education programs. The Council on Continuing Medical Education approves programs and credits for continuing medical education. The Council on International Osteopathic Medical Education and Affairs address international training concerns. Osteopathic graduate training is organized around community-based training consortia, known as Osteopathic Postdoctoral Training Institutions. These consortia consist of at least one medical school accredited by AOA and several hospitals that are accredited by AOA's Bureau of Health Facilities' Accreditation (see www.aacom.org)

Nursing education: Accreditation of nursing programs is provided by two groups. One is the National League for Nursing Accrediting Commission (NLNAC), an independent entity within the National League for Nursing. NLNAC accredits all types of nursing programs, from the diploma through the doctoral level (National League for Nursing Accreditation Commission, 2001). The other is the Commission on Collegiate Nursing Education (CCNE), established by the American Association of Colleges of Nursing. CCNE focuses only on nursing programs in universities and 4-year colleges (American Association of Colleges of Nursing, 2002c), providing accreditation services for programs at the baccalaureate and graduate degree levels. Accreditation for programs for nurse practitioners is also becoming standardized, although four different groups will have unique certifying exams (Phillips et al., 2002).

Public health education: Schools of public health, community health education programs, and community health/preventive medicine programs are accredited by the Council on Education for Public Health (Council on Education for Public Health, 2002). The Council is a private, nonprofit organization with two members: the American Public Health Association and the Association of Schools of Public Health. The primary professional degree is the Master of Public Health (MPH), but other master's and doctoral degrees are offered as well.

Health Administration: The Accrediting Commission on Education for Health Services Administration (ACEHSA) is the organization authorized by the U.S. Department of Education to accredit master's level health administration programs in the United States and Canada. Graduate programs in health care administration are housed in various schools and departments on university campuses. These programs are found in schools of business, medicine, public health, public administration, and allied health sciences, as well as schools of graduate studies. The degrees awarded by these programs include MA, MBA, MHA, MHSA, MPH, MS, and others (Accrediting Commission on Education for Health Services Administration, 2001).

the purposes of continuing education is to supplement areas in which undergraduate or graduate training has been deficient (Waxman and Kimball, 1999), such information should be provided systematically to those education programs so the deficiencies can be addressed. The current fragmentation inhibits these interactions. A recent Institute of Medicine report (2003a) calls on all education oversight organizations (accrediting, licensing, and certifying bodies) to work together to revise their standards.

Faculty Development and Organization

The school and its faculty are the strongest influences on the design of curriculum and students' educational experiences. Accrediting groups define standards for the structure, performance, and/or functions of the schools, but do not prescribe specific courses or educational experiences. The latter is the responsibility of each school as it designs its own curriculum within the guidelines of the pertinent oversight bodies. Even with a bounty of standards, it is known that schools vary in terms of emphasis, resources, costs, size, centralized or decentralized curriculum, frequency of curricular change, and other factors.

Faculty are being asked to assume new duties in areas in which they may not be adequately prepared to teach the next generation. Faculty teaching today may themselves not have been trained in nonhospital settings, computer-based systems, or interdisciplinary approaches to care (Wilkerson and Irby, 1998). They may not have learned how to develop curricula, evaluate students, or manage educational programs (Gelmon, 1996). Most medical teaching occurs through one-on-one encounters between physician and patient, reflecting the comfort level and expertise of many faculty (Kaufman, 1999). As a result, faculty may be unsure about their own skills for implementing aspects of a new curriculum (Sachdeva, 2000). Being a knowledgeable clinician (or basic scientist) does not necessarily translate to being an effective teacher.

There are also concerns about the availability of faculty in terms of both supply and time. As noted earlier, teaching faculty are under pressure to see patients and conduct research, leaving little time for teaching (The Commonwealth Fund Task Force on Academic Health Centers, 2002; Ludmerer, 1999). Although this concern is often voiced about medical faculty, it has been suggested that as nursing practice plans develop, a similar pattern will ensue. Nursing faculty will also face constraints on time for teaching as the pressure to see patients and raise revenue increases (Conway-Welch, 2002). Furthermore, particularly in nursing, there are concerns about the adequacy of the supply of faculty (American Association of Colleges of Nursing, 2002b; Association of Academic Health Centers, 2002).

The pressures on faculty preparation and time are likely to intensify as training is expanded to encompass a range of sites. More faculty with more-varied backgrounds could enhance the educational experience for students but could also result in even greater variability in student training. Faculty development will be needed to ensure that the faculty available at all training sites are prepared to teach students effectively (Weed, 1981; Griner and Danoff, 2000). Some have suggested using a smaller, full-time faculty (Hanft, 1988), perhaps moving with the students rather than the clinicians in each site taking on faculty duties.

In medical schools, the decentralized structure of faculty with powerful department chairs is viewed as a force that can inhibit educational innovation (Cantor et al., 1991; Regan-Smith, 1998; Petersdorf and Turner, 1995). Faculty identify predominantly with their own department and focus on training in their own discipline, hindering a broad, integrated view of clinical education. The strong departmental structure can also make it difficult to incorporate broad-based education courses that are not departmentally defined; for example, population health or "evaluative" sciences, such as biostatistics or epidemiology. Some schools have moved toward a more centralized curriculum to overcome the problems of a departmentally organized model, and although improvements are seen in terms of curricular reform, they also tend to raise costs because of the increased time needed for faculty coordination (Reynolds et al., 1995).

Weak Evidence Base

The evidence base for clinical education is not as strong as it should be to support the reforms described in this chapter. Better information is needed on the effectiveness of various teaching approaches for clinicians, on how principles of adult education can be applied appropriately to clinical education, on what types of teaching technologies are most effective and under what circumstances, on the characteristics associated with high-quality clinical education, and on the cost of training various health professionals. Good quality measures in clinical education do not currently exist (Blumenthal and Bass, 2001).

The Cochrane Collaboration has been working for many years to develop the evidence base for clinical care, but there is no comparable resource for the evidence base in clinical education. When the Cochrane Collaboration attempted to conduct a systematic review of educational interventions for teaching evidence-based medicine, only one article was found that met their criteria for inclusion (Hatala and Guyatt, 2002).

Two relatively new groups are making such an effort at developing an evidence base. The Campbell Collaboration (formally established in 2000) prepares and maintains systematic reviews of the effects of social and education policies and practices (see www.campbellcollaboration.org). For example, a systematic review is being prepared for problem-based learning for health professionals (Davies and Boruch, 2001). The second group, Best Evidence Medical Education, is a collaboration of individuals and organizations committed to the dissemination of information to people involved in medical education; the production of systematic reviews of medical education; and the creation of a culture of best-evidence medical education among teachers, institutions, and national bodies (see www.bemecollaboration.org). The group has been meeting since 1999. Both groups are international, with a strong European representation.

There is also a lack of information on the actual cost of education programs and its relationship to the quality of education (Henderson, 2000). Spending patterns for public funds are known, but how much training costs is not understood. Medicare payment per resident is known to vary, but it is believed to reflect historical accounting practices rather than true differences in the cost or quality of programs (Young and Coffman, 1998). Many schools have not budgeted systematically for clinical education (The Commonwealth Fund Task Force on Academic Health Centers, 2002). Because current information is so poor, it is difficult to estimate the costs for educational reform or identify areas in which savings might occur (The Commonwealth Fund Task Force on Academic Health Centers, 2002). For example, costs might be incurred to implement computer-based instruction, but could reduce faculty time in some areas.

Financing

As discussed in more detail in Chapter 6, current financing methods for clinical education are not viewed as being supportive of the types of changes advocated in this report (LeRoy, 1994). The current methods have encouraged increases in the number, size, and duration of residency programs (Henderson, 1999, 2000) and programs for the training of specialists in tertiary settings (Young and Coffman, 1998). These methods have also hindered training in nonhospital settings (Henderson, 2000). Moreover, funding is not linked to any workforce goals, whether they be the types of changes described here or other goals related to the supply and mix of the output of the programs.

Interdisciplinary training is also discouraged by variation in how the education of different professions is supported. When Medicare began, educational costs for nursing and allied health professionals were allowable expenses for hospitals. Since 1965, however, many hospital-based training programs have been eliminated. For example, in 1965, 80 percent of training programs for registered nurses were in hospital-operated programs;

today the figure is only 7 percent (Medicare Payment Advisory Commission, 2001). Medicare currently supports diploma nursing programs, programs for nurse anesthetists, and training for allied health professionals that are hospital-based programs. About one-half of hospitals with residency training programs also receive money for nursing and allied health training (Medicare Payment Advisory Commission, 2001). However, AHCs offer few hospital-based training programs, so the training support provided for medicine and that for nursing and allied health are going to different organizations, discouraging an interdisciplinary perspective. Another difference is that services provided jointly by a medical resident and supervising physician may be reimbursed, whereas the same is not true for other students. Therefore, nonmedical students do not offer the same advantages in cost recovery to the hospital sponsoring a training program; the result, again, is an emphasis on medicine.

IMPLICATIONS FOR THE FUTURE

There have been many calls for reform of clinical education, especially medical education. A recent Institute of Medicine report (2003a) urges an overhaul in health professions education. Likewise, in their survey of medical school deans, Cantor, et al. (1991) found that 68 percent believed fundamental change was needed in medical education. This was true for their own institutions, as well as for medical education overall. Petersdorf and Turner (1995, p. 541) report that the education given to students is "dated and arcane" and not in tune with societal needs. In interpreting their survey of young physicians, Cantor et al. (1993, p. 1035) find that "while medical training has remained largely unchanged, the demands placed on practicing physicians have changed dramatically." At a workshop sponsored by the committee during the course of this study, Hundert (2002) described the current process of medical education as one that can "take altruistic other-oriented people and turn them into bitter cynics, in four short years."

The current curriculum is perceived as overcrowded and relying too much on memorization of facts, and the changes implemented have not altered the underlying experience of educators and students (Regan-Smith, 1998). Current processes of education are too static and passive and do not focus sufficiently on teaching students how to solve real, everyday problems and measure the effectiveness of interventions through such sciences as epidemiology, informatics, health services research, and outcomes analysis (Detmer 1997). The fundamental approach to clinical education has not changed since 1910, or as some have observed, there has been "reform without change" (Christakis, 1995, p. 710). Others have gone so far as to suggest that the current model of education is so mismatched with today's complex health care environment that a "drastic overhaul" is needed (Chassin, 1998, p. 579).

AHCs will need to provide leadership in effecting the broad educational reforms required to prepare health professionals to meet the needs of the 21st century health system. Most educational reform to date has taken the approach of overlaying courses on the existing curriculum and structure. The result has been the overcrowded curriculum noted earlier, wide variation across programs, and poor progress in some areas. What is needed is more comprehensive and fundamental reform of the educational experience that spans the continuum of education and recognizes the shifting roles and responsibilities among health professionals, along with the interactions of those shifts.

In taking up this challenge, AHCs will need to work more closely with their parent universities, using the academic and interdisciplinary resources available. Schools of education should be consulted in the development of educational methodology. Coordination of basic science and social science courses in the university should be explored in an effort to streamline the education process and foster interactions among faculty at different schools. Interdisciplinary approaches should work in both directions. University students in engineering or computational biology should have the opportunity to conduct work at the AHC; exposure to such work could interest them in applying their much-needed skills to health care. Similarly, students at the AHC should be encouraged to explore the resources available throughout the university, such as at a business or law school.

Public policy also needs to support changes in education that respond to changes in health care. Policy makers need to consider how financing methods can support both short- and long-term changes in clinical education. Innovative approaches are especially needed in implementing methods to support interdisciplinary education, and to provide training in information management, as well as in developing nonhospital training sites.

CHAPTER 4

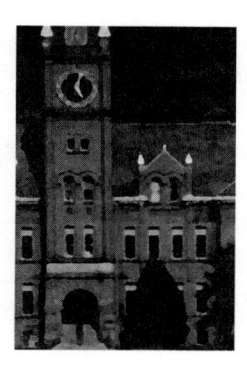

THE ACADEMIC HEALTH CENTER AS A MODELER: THE PATIENT CARE ROLE

At a workshop sponsored by the committee during the course of this study, Snyderman (2002) coined the term "service platform" to denote the need for a better model of care delivery capable of exploiting the new technologies and capabilities that will characterize the health care system of the future. In the words of another workshop participant, "we are trying to put a new genotype on an old phenotype." It is necessary to redesign the processes of care, but doing so will also require altering the structures that deliver care.

The term "platform" has been used in other industries. In information technology, it denotes the infrastructure that permits a particular use or analysis of information. In the military, the term refers to the ways in which workforce, equipment, and organization should be arranged to produce a specific capability or response. In both of these cases, the platform is designed to produce a clear output. Rather than starting from the available capabilities and determining what can be done, designers first ask what needs to be done and then design the platform to deliver it.

This same concept can be applied in considering how to design a new service platform for health care. Given the trends described in the Chapter 2, those who deliver health care need to ask how current models for and approaches to care can be redesigned not only to treat the illnesses of patients but also to improve the health of patients and populations. If health care is to produce a different output, the platform for delivering that output needs to be rethought. In examining the clinical care role of AHCs, the committee finds the following:

- AHCs are major providers of specialty care, and many also provide significant levels of care to the poor and uninsured. AHCs therefore have a dual safety net role as provider of last resort for the critically ill, and for the poor and uninsured.
- AHCs need to play a part in redesigning care if they are to respond to the changing demands that will arise in the coming decades and be able to deliver the improved capabilities that the system will have the potential to offer.
- The clinical care setting is where the AHC research and education roles intersect. The ability to incorporate the new sciences developed by research into care delivery and successfully teach students how to practice in the evolving environment of care will depend on how effectively AHCs can adapt their clinical care settings.

The first section below examines the need for new models of care. The next two sections review the contributions of AHCs to patient care and the challenges facing AHCs as they work to design better models of care. The final section presents some implications for the future.

THE NEED FOR NEW MODELS OF CARE

The shifts and developments that will occur in health care over the coming decades argue strongly for the creation of new approaches to the organization and delivery of care. Better models are needed for care for the chronically ill and for use of the latest information and biomedical technologies to maximize both the quality of care and the cost-effectiveness.

Current models of care are heavily focused on interventions for treating illness. There is evidence that better approaches are needed to improve health. Although mortality rates have declined across all age groups, these general declines mask important differences (Institute of Medicine, 2002d). For example, lung cancer and chronic respiratory disease have declined or remained stable for men but increased for women (National Center for Health Statistics, 2002). Likewise, differences by race have been identified in both the diagnosis and use of therapeutic procedures for cardiovascular care (Lurie and Buntin, 2002). Since cardiovascular disease is one of the leading causes of death in the United States, improving care for those afflicted could have a significant impact if designed and targeted properly (Wong et al., 2002). As noted earlier in this report, chronic illness is the leading cause of illness and disability among the U.S. population, yet too many of those affected do not recieve adequate treatment (Wagner et al., 1996), including guidance on lifestyle changes that can help in preventing and managing these conditions.

In addition, as noted above, care delivery exhibits variations that are unrelated to type or severity of illness or patient preferences (Wennberg, 2002). The risk of hospitalization at all of Boston's teaching hospitals is higher than that at Yale–New Haven Hospital, even after adjusting for age, sex, race, illness, and the price of medical care (Center for the Evaluative Clinical Sciences at Dartmouth Medical School, 1999a). Among referral areas that contain at least one medical school, the age-, sex-, race-, and illness-adjusted discharge rate for medical conditions per 1,000 Medicare enrollees ranges from 285 in Jackson, Mississippi, to 165 in Salt Lake City (Center for the Evaluative Clinical Sciences at Dartmouth Medical School, 1999b). Medicare beneficiaries who live in regions that exhibit higher spending levels receive about 60 percent more care than residents in lower-spending regions but do not show better quality of care, outcomes, or satisfaction with care (Fisher et al., 2003). Some variation would be expected and desirable to reflect patient preferences and customized care. However, the levels of variation among all institutions across the country (not just AHCs) suggest that much of clinical practice remains empirical and not necessarily driven by science (Wennberg, 2002).

In general, current approaches to care are reactive, involving treating patients when they present with symptoms through a series of sporadic interventions that are predominantly physician directed. To address the changing needs of people and exploit technological advances, 21st century health care will need to be more proactive, interactive with patients, and evidence based (Snyderman and Saito, 2000). The prevalence of chronic illness will demand better approaches to care, and the new technologies will enable the prediction and prevention of disease, especially through an understanding of genetic susceptibility and behavioral risks and the benefits of their modification.

Examples of better models of care are beginning to emerge. These models target particular populations, such as those with chronic illness, the frail elderly, the poor, the uninsured, and those with specific conditions. The examples described here are offered as illustrative examples to demonstrate that better approaches are possible.

The Chronic Care Model is designed to improve coordination and collaboration in care for chronically ill populations. The model is characterized by (1) a protocol or plan containing an explicit description of what is to be done for individual patients, as well as for groups of patients with specific clinical features; (2) a redesign of practice to include regular patient contact, collection of data on health and disease status, and efforts to address patients' psychosocial needs; (3) a strong focus on patient information and self-management, including support for behavioral and lifestyle changes to improve outcomes of care; (4) the availability of specialized expertise for practitioners managing care; and (5) good information about patients, their care, and the outcomes of care, including the use of registries and reminder systems to support care plans (Wagner et al., 1996). The model emphasizes self-management, care planning with an interdisciplinary team, ongoing assessment and follow-up, and linkages with community programs (e.g., exercise programs) (Bodenheimer et al., 2002; Institute of Medicine, 2001b; Lurie and Buntin, 2002). Although care for the chronically ill demands greater coordination and communication along the continuum of care settings, the current system is characterized by fragmentation and poor coordination. For instance, it has been estimated that fewer than half of patients with hypertension, depression, diabetes, and asthma are receiving appropriate treatment (Rundall et al., 2002).

A second model, focused on the frail elderly, is the Program for All-Inclusive Care for the Elderly, or PACE. This model is designed to provide and coordinate all needed preventive, primary, acute, and long-term care for the frail elderly, with the aim of optimizing health and functioning while permitting participants in the program to continue to live in the community (Program of All Inclusive Care for the Elderly, 2002). The program was developed during the 1970s, was tested beginning in the 1980s, and was established as a permanent model in Medicare under the Balanced Budget Act of 1997. Evaluations of PACE programs have found that participants have better functional status, receive more primary care and preventive services, and experience fewer days in the hospital despite having greater morbidity and disability than other elderly populations, although programs exhibited considerable variation (Burton et al., 2002; Wieland et al., 2000; Mukamel et al., 1998). A number of AHCs, including Johns Hopkins, Mount Sinai, and the University of Pennsylvania, sponsor PACE programs, (Program of All Inclusive Care for the Elderly, 2002).

Better models of care can also result in improved care for poor and uninsured populations. The University of New Mexico, for example, created a type of managed care arrangement for the uninsured. This model emphasized primary care, a continuous patient–physician relationship, and the priority of preventive care (Kaufman et al., 2000). Results observed over a 2-year period revealed that ambulatory visits (including those to the emergency room), hospital discharges, and hospital days decreased. Among the subset of high users, outpatient and specialty visits increased, hospital discharges and days decreased, and there was no change in the number of emergency room visits. Hospital revenues increased as well because the lost volume was replaced by paying patients. Meeting the needs of this population also required attention to social support services, such as transportation, translation, and other types of referrals (e.g., to literacy programs). Prior to this program, the emphasis was on providing inpatient and specialty services for primary care problems, which did not meet the needs of this group (Kaufman et al., 2000).

The Diabetes Control and Complications Trial represents the development of an intensive care strategy to care for people with diabetes. Sponsored by the National Institute of Diabetes and Digestive and Kidney Diseases from 1983 to 1993 and conducted in multiple sites, the study showed that the onset and progression of complications from diabetes could be slowed with intensive clinical management that included not only testing of blood glucose levels four or more times a day, four daily insulin injections (or use of an insulin pump), and adjustment of insulin doses according to food intake and exercise, but also a diet and exercise plan and monthly visits to a health care team that included a physician, nurse educator, dietitian, and behavioral therapist (National Institute of Diabetes and Digestive and Kidney Diseases, 2002). Effective management required a clear and explicit clinical plan, strong patient involvement, and the support of an integrated care team. This approach is similar to disease management models that emphasize a systematic approach to care, employ interdisciplinary teams to deliver care, use practice guidelines and protocols appropriate to the target population, and can potentially include services across the entire continuum of care (Blumenthal and Buntin, 1998).

A report of the Institute of Medicine (2001b)—*Crossing the Quality Chasm: A New Health System for the 21st Century*—describes the need for redesigning care delivery in several areas. First, the processes used to deliver care need to be made more reliable and to make better use of information technologies to automate clinical information and improve communications. Second, clinicians must be provided with the new knowledge they will need to translate the evidence base into practice and manage the resulting changes. Third, interdisciplinary teams must be created and maintained; to this end, it will be necessary to overcome training, structural, and financial barriers that can hinder team functioning. Fourth, care needs to be better coordinated across patient conditions, services, and settings and over time; coordination with community resources or the public health system is particularly difficult to achieve. Finally, performance and outcome measures for improvement and accountability need to be incorporated into the daily work of health care organizations so they can continually evaluate and improve the care delivered.

Several characteristics are common across the models described above. First, each encompasses an interdisciplinary approach. As discussed earlier, interdisciplinary teams are needed in health care, in part because of the increased complexity of care. Treatment for many conditions is so complex that the knowledge of multiple practitioners—including various medical specialists as well as other clinicians, such as therapists or nutritionists—is needed to manage a single condition. In addition, there has been a significant increase in the number of nonphysician clinicians. In the early 1900s, physicians represented one of every three health care workers (Aiken, 2001). Today this figure is about one in ten (counting health practitioners involved in direct care, and excluding managers and support personnel) (Bureau of Labor Statistics, 2001). As the mix of health care workers diversifies, they must increasingly work in teams to deliver care. Characteristics of effective teams include appropriate size and composition, good communication processes, clarity in team tasks, and an environment in which the team can acquire needed resources (Institute of Medicine, 2001b). Ineffective teams can inadvertently cause errors if, for example, there are too many hand-offs that are not well planned or executed properly. The field of aviation is often cited as a model for the training and attention given to developing effective teams (Institute of Medicine, 2000).

A second common characteristic of the models described above is a patient-centered focus. Patient-centered care is defined as "health care that is closely congruent with and responsive to patients' wants, needs and preferences" (Laine and Davidoff, 1996, p. 152). It encompasses disclosure of information to and active discourse with patients; patients' participation in decision making about their care; and recognition of outcomes that include functional status, satisfaction, and quality, all of which require patient input to measure.

Patient-centered care is assuming increasing importance for a variety of reasons. For one thing, chronic illness demands greater self-management by patients (Bodenheimer et al., 2002). For another, as technological advances expand treatment options, the choice of treatment should reflect patient input when possible and desired by the patient (Barry et al., 1995). There is also evidence that patients who are more involved in their care have better outcomes (Institute of Medicine, 2003b). Finally, there is some evidence that patients who share in decision making may have decreased demand for services (Wagner et al., 1995). Therefore, redesigned models of care need to recognize the patient as part of the care-giving team.

Finally, all of the models described above are characterized by a broad view of health that not only reflects excellent science-based clinical care but also addresses other factors that influence health, such as exercise, nutrition counseling, and community services. The models were designed to revolve around the needs of patients to maximize their health and functioning, instead of focusing on the capabilities of a particular setting of care.

CONTRIBUTIONS OF AHCS TO PATIENT CARE

AHCs are recognized throughout the world for their specialty care. Although AHC hospitals represent just 3 percent of all hospitals in the United States, they house 33 percent of transplant services, 16 percent of neonatal units, and 15 percent of open-heart surgical units (see Appendix A). The provision of specialty services at AHCs also ensures standby capacity that benefits the local community. Like fire departments, AHCs assure people that the services of a trauma or burn unit are available.

About half of patients with rare and uncommon conditions are cared for at AHCs and major teaching hospitals. Yet such patients represent a relatively small proportion of the volume at these centers, accounting for about 13 percent of overall admissions (The Commonwealth Fund Task Force on Academic Health Centers, 2000), although individual AHCs may exhibit differing proportions of routine to specialty care. AHCs also receive a large proportion of patients who are transferred from other hospitals for all types of care (not just rare and uncommon conditions). The Commonwealth Task Force on Academic Health Centers (2000) estimates that the proportion of AHC patients who were transferred from other hospitals was more than 8 percent in 1995, up from about 5 percent 3 years earlier. Transfer patients tend to be older, to have more comorbidities, and to require more complex treatment than other patients.

The AHC clinical enterprise has grown rapidly in recent years. Overall, the average daily census at AHC hospitals has declined by 2 percent between 1990 and 2000, but during the same period, outpatient volume has increased by 133 percent; emergency room visits by 54 percent (see Appendix A); and clinical faculty, who deliver the care, by 52 percent (Jonas et al., 1990; Barzansky and Etzel, 2001). In 1990, AHCs represented 2 percent of hospitals, 7 percent of hospital beds, and 10 percent of total hospital days; by 1999, they represented 3 percent of hospitals, 10 percent of hospital beds, and 13 percent of total hospital days (see Appendix A). The market share of AHC hospitals increased during a time at which inpatient admissions in general were declining. For most AHCs, revenues from clinical activities support education and research activities and make it possible to care for the uninsured. Whether these historical levels of growth can be sustained into the future is unclear, however.

As discussed earlier, many AHCs are also an important part of their local community's safety net. In a study of 38 communities with AHCs (Reuter, 1999), the AHCs represented about 6 percent of hospitals and 13 percent of hospital beds, yet they provided:

- 36 percent of care for Medicaid AIDS patients and 34 percent of uninsured AIDS patients.
- 36 percent of trauma care for Medicaid trauma cases and 36 percent of uninsured trauma cases.
- 25 percent of care for Medicaid high-risk infants and 26 percent of care for uninsured high-risk infants.

Although there has been much analysis of safety-net providers, The Commonwealth Task Force on Academic Health Centers is one of the few sources that has specifically examined AHCs (as opposed to teaching hospitals or hospitals generally). The task force has estimated that in 1991, AHC hospitals accounted for almost 40 percent of total charity care provided; by 1996, this proportion had grown to 44 percent (The Commonwealth Fund Task Force on Academic Health Centers, 2001). During the same period, the number of uninsured patients cared for at AHC hospitals grew from 20 to 28 percent. Moreover, care for the uninsured appears to be growing as a proportion of all care provided at AHCs. In terms of hospital costs, uncompensated care was estimated at 7 percent of costs at AHCs in 2000, an increase of almost 2 percentage points since 1994 as compared with a 1 percent increase for other hospitals (Dobson et al., 2002).

Public AHCs appear to play a larger safety-net role than private AHCs. The Commonwealth Task Force found that of the total charity care provided in 1996, 31 percent was provided by public AHC hospitals and 13 percent by private AHC hospitals, a pattern similar to that exhibited by public and private hospitals generally (The Commonwealth Task Force on Academic Health Centers, 2001). In the previously noted study of 38 communities with AHCs, public AHC hospitals treated 17 percent of all uninsured and 10 percent of all Medicaid patients in those markets, whereas private AHC hospitals treated 5 percent of all uninsured and just over 7 percent of all Medicaid patients (Reuter, 1999).

A number of factors influence the safety-net role of AHCs. As noted above, public ownership is one factor. Geographic location is another, with many AHCs being located in central cities where large numbers of poor and uninsured people reside. It may be noted that the AHC safety net role has supported clinical education by providing students with a volume of patients for their training experiences.

A major source of support for hospitals that serve large numbers of poor people is disproportionate-share funds provided by Medicare and some state governments. According to figures presented to the committee, Medicare disproportionate-share funds are highly dispersed, going to approximately 4,000 institutions, only some of which are AHCs (Anderson, 2002). One of the main concerns regarding disproportionate-share funding is that the formula does not adequately target hospitals that serve the greatest numbers of poor and uninsured (see Chapter 6). Furthermore, by paying for hospital care, the arrangement does not encourage the development of better models of care that are more responsive to the needs of these populations (such as the University of New Mexico example described earlier in this chapter).

According to recent evidence, AHC hospitals that serve more poor and uninsured people have lower financial margins than other hospitals. In 2000, the aggregate total margin for public AHC hospitals declined to –3.7 percent (–6.7 percent for aggregate operating margins), whereas total margins for private AHC hospitals increased to the 1998 level of 4.4 percent (1.1 percent for aggregate operating margins) (Dobson et al., 2002).

The concern is that safety-net AHCs may have fewer resources and options available to them relative to other hospitals (Zuckerman et al., 2001). Although the implementation of information technology could produce efficiencies that are needed by safety-net providers in particular, pursuing such a strategy requires capital investment. Similarly, redesigning care will require working capital and could result in temporarily higher operating costs as the organization transitions to new programs and operating designs. There is also concern about access by the poor and uninsured. Hospitals (including those at AHCs) that are facing reductions in revenues generally seek ways to become more efficient but may also limit access for medically indigent patients (The Kaiser Family Foundation, 2001).

CHALLENGES TO AHCS IN DESIGNING BETTER MODELS OF CARE

The pressures to redesign models of care can be expected to increase. As noted earlier, the shifts in the needs of the population and changing composition of the workforce will necessitate better approaches to care. Furthermore, as noted in Chapter 2, the increased demand for care brought about the aging population, combined with a slow growth in the size of the labor force, can be expected to result in increased labor costs, along with demands for productivity improvements. Labor shortages, such as in nursing, will add to the pressures to redesign care.

AHCs have an important role to play in redesigning models of care for at least four reasons. First, as part of the direct care delivery system, AHCs need to ensure that they are providing care designed to meet patients' needs and improve health. As noted earlier in this chapter, well-designed processes of care affect the health of patients.

Second, through their research role, AHCs create the knowledge that drives the care received by patients. Part of translating that knowledge into practice is understanding and improving the organizational context in which the care is delivered. A research scientist may develop a procedure or other element of care that is technically sound, but if it is delivered through a poor design, its full benefits may not be realized. AHCs need to redesign care so that new knowledge discovered can also be delivered.

Third, the care provided at AHCs needs to demonstrate evidence-based best practices for the students who are learning in these settings. Students should be taught to practice models of care that are designed to improve health. Therefore, it is important that AHCs view the clinical care setting as one component of their academic activities and use it to develop, test, refine, and improve processes of care.

Fourth, AHCs need to ensure a good working environment within their own organizations to attract and retain a high-quality workforce. For example, one factor contributing to the current nursing shortage is dissatisfaction with the work environment, including a lack of respect, a lack of recognition, a lack of participation in decision making, and an erosion of the nurse–patient relationship (Association of Academic Health Centers, 2002b). Since labor represents about half of a hospital's operating expenses (Sochalski et al., 1997), redesigning care to improve the health of patients will also require examining work processes and the use of human resources.

AHCs are recognized for technological innovation, but they are not automatically associated with organizational innovation. Many of the efforts undertaken to date to reorganize care and people have involved "reengineering," or the simultaneous restructuring of work processes and organizational design (Walston et al., 2000). Reengineering reallocates and readjusts work flows and job responsibilities, and determines where work is located, who does the work, and how the work will get done. Reengineering efforts in health care generally have not lived up to their promise, however. Efforts have typically been based in departments, and have thus failed to address overall issues of organizational design (Aiken, 2001). For example, it may not be possible to resolve issues related to nurses' dissatisfaction with the work environment at the departmental level. Hospitals found to be more successful in attracting and retaining nurses are characterized by a professional practice environment that fosters greater autonomy for nurses, their greater control over support services, and better communication between physicians and nurses (Steinbrook, 2002; Aiken, 2002).

As discussed earlier, another challenge facing AHCs is the need to make greater investments in information and communications technology for monitoring and evaluating care, and for understanding the relationship between processes of care and outcomes. Assessing patterns of care for groups of patients will demand better information technology that can aggregate data across the patient's experience, especially across settings and over time. Information and communications technology can also serve as glue that holds care teams together, getting information to people whenever and wherever it is needed. In one example, the University of California (UC) system is installing a Web-based medical-event reporting system to improve patient safety in its medical centers and provide a means for rapid identification of areas for improvement (University of California, 2003). This is the first effort of its type, linking five AHCs—UC Davis, UC Irvine, UC Los Angeles, UC San Francisco, and UC San Diego—on a systemwide basis through the Internet, permitting front-line clinical workers to report on adverse and near-miss events from most computers in each of the participating medical centers. The system includes the establishment of a severity ranking to permit comparisons within and across campuses. Monthly conferences will be held to address findings.

IMPLICATIONS FOR THE FUTURE

AHCs need to develop the structures, processes, and team approaches necessary to achieve improvements in health for the patients and populations that rely on them. Asking AHCs to redesign care will mean requiring that they conceptualize new models of care. This is different from improving or refining a particular technique or procedure, for example. Although those aspects of care need to be developed and do produce improvements in care, conceptualizing new models of care will require AHCs to describe, design, and shape new approaches to care that are patient-centered and aimed at improving health. Some envision a more proactive model of care that identifies people at risk of major disease and intervenes early to prospectively alter the progression of disease (Williams et al., 2003). Conceptually, interventions could include customized care that relies on the latest biomedical advances, but also community interventions aimed at specific subpopulations.

Given the patient populations served by most AHCs, redesign should focus in particular on people at high risk for serious illness and those who are financially vulnerable. Redesign should also emphasize methods for encouraging patient self-management and adoption of healthy behaviors. Achieving such redesign will require that AHCs work across all of their component organizations, including nursing schools and public schools and programs, as well as with their local communities.

Implementing new models of care will also require delivery system changes that include greater reliance on information systems, patient self-management that necessitates expanded health education and support, a team orientation, and decision support (Berenson and Horvath, 2003). However, current payment methods create several obstacles to making these types of delivery changes.

First, the types of services that are most focused on improving and maintaining health are not as well supported by payers as medical services. For example, patient education for self-management is supported by Medicare in only limited circumstances, such as diabetes care (Berenson and Horvath, 2003).

Second, current methods have weak or no incentives to improve care or health, and are generally not designed to support coordination of care, interdisciplinary team approaches to care, or improvements in health. Fee-for-service payment rewards the delivery of individual units of care, an arrangement that inhibits coordination and team approaches and rewards treatment of illness (Institute of Medicine, 2001b). Providers focus on their own activities and functions without attention to the effect on costs or care across settings or providers (Berenson and Horvath, 2003).

Third, providers can lose money by improving care. For example, a pilot project at Duke University improved outcomes of care and reduced annual expenses by almost 40 percent for patients with congestive heart failure. However, Duke lost money because patients stayed out of the hospital, avoiding procedures that are relatively well reimbursed, while incurring greater expenses for ambulatory care and patient education, which are more poorly reimbursed (Williams et al., 2003). In another example, a physician group that was paid through fee-for-services methods improved care for diabetes patients and achieved cost savings through reduced visits and hospitalizations but lost money in two ways (Institute of Medicine, 2001b). First, they incurred the expenses for tighter clinical management that produced the improved outcomes. Second, the savings due to reduced hospitalizations and visits accrued to the insurer rather than the provider that had made the savings possible. Providers cannot be expected to sustain care improvements if they will predictably lose money for doing so.

Capitation payment arrangements should provide greater flexibility to coordinate care and allocate resources according to the needs of patient groups but appear to be diminishing as a payment method (Hurley et al., 2002). Furthermore, capitation arrangements may be narrowly defined, covering only office visits or ambulatory care, for example, rather than a comprehensive continuum of care that would be required under a chronic care or other model (Dudley and Luft, 2001). Shared-risk arrangements may offer a stronger potential for both payers and providers to gain from care improvements and cost savings. However, such arrangements would likely require a partnership between the payer and provider, as well as longer-term contracts to permit the needed investments and make it possible to obtain the rewards of the improvements, rather than the annual arrangements most typical today (Institute of Medicine, 2001b).

Redesigning care to improve health is not the responsibility of AHCs or of payers and employers—it is the responsibility of all. AHCs should help guide payers and policy makers with regard to the characteristics of care models that improve health for patients and populations and the features that best demonstrate evidence-based, continuously improving, cost-efficient practice, recognizing that payers and employers have to balance the cost *and* quality *and* access needs of a population of enrollees and beneficiaries. Payers and employees should support demonstration projects that aim to build better models of care, recognizing the priorities of the other. Payers need to recognize that redesigning care will require some experimentation, that not all plans will work as designed, and that there is a cost for testing new approaches while not abandoning the status quo (in essence, maintaining dual systems).

CHAPTER 5

THE ACADEMIC HEALTH CENTER AS A TRANSLATOR OF SCIENCE: THE RESEARCH ROLE

Advances in health care in the 20th century, especially those emerging from basic research, were remarkable. The mapping of the human genome in particular is expected to have a profound effect on the future of health care (Pober et al., 2001). Many believe that in the 21st century, the life sciences will emulate the intellectual and economic feats of the physical sciences in the last century (Greenberg, 2000). Expectations are high that the burden of disease and disability can be reduced through research.

As we embark on the 21st century, it is important to maintain the capacity for continued discovery in the basic sciences. Without a greater focus on clinical, health services, and prevention research, however, the full benefits of such discoveries will not be realized. Research provides the foundation for our current scientific knowledge; the challenge in the future will be to translate that knowledge and the resulting expanded capabilities into daily practice (Frist, 2002). This chapter examines how the research role of AHCs can be used to improve the health of people and develop the scientific evidence base for health and health care. Overall, the committee finds the following:

- AHCs have been significant contributors to the enormous strides made by research in the past decades, especially those of basic scientific research. Investments in basic science should be continued to support advances in discovery and understanding. AHCs and their parent universities play a critical role in the long-term basic research that makes future innovations possible.

- In the coming decades, continued scientific discoveries and advances will require that AHCs continue their work in basic science research and discovery, as well as developing and refining the evidence base for health care by:
  — Encouraging studies that embrace the continuum from animals to humans to experimental models.
  — Increasing the emphasis on clinical research in order to translate new discoveries into clinical practice and evaluate current clinical practices, thereby answering questions about what does and does not work in health care.
  — Increasing emphasis on health services research in order to improve understanding of the effectiveness and costs of care, especially the impact of new discoveries on the costs of care and treatment patterns.
  — Increasing emphasis on prevention and population research in order to improve understanding of how to identify and reduce health risks, as well as the linkages between personal and population health.

This chapter describes the continuum of research and the challenges that will be faced in the coming decades by both AHCs and the agencies that fund health-related research. The first section examines the processes by which the scientific evidence base for health is created and applied. The next two sections, respectively, review the continuum of research from discovery through application and the obstacles faced by AHCs in conducting research across this continuum. The final section presents some implications for the future.

CREATING AND APPLYING THE SCIENTIFIC EVIDENCE BASE FOR HEALTH

The trends and shifts described in Chapter 2 will create both opportunities and challenges for research in the coming decades. The rapid pace of discovery will generate opportunities to improve health in new and potentially more effective ways. Advances in the past have yielded great benefits in terms of outcomes of care, increased longevity, improved quality of life, and reduced absenteeism from work (Cutler and McClellan, 2001). Illnesses once thought to be incurable can now be treated, and sometimes cured or prevented, as a result of the scientific and technological advances made possible by basic research (Frist, 2002).

Many believe that science is on the cusp of generating a major revolution in medicine as a result of advances in genomics, proteomics, and such areas as stem cell biology that offer the potential for new breakthroughs in tissue engineering. One researcher suggests we are "at the beginning of the end" of a phase of discovery that involves identifying the molecules required for human life (Pollard, 2002, p. 1725). Most molecular defects are seen at the cellular, organ, or organismic level. Current knowledge is linking an individual's predisposition to disease, but additional understanding of the underlying mechanisms will be needed to move toward preventive medicine at the molecular level (Pollard, 2002). It is also now feasible to conduct studies in humans that were not possible in the past, potentially improving understanding of the pathogenesis of disease. More proof-of-concept studies in human subjects are needed if new diagnostic and therapeutic approaches are to emerge from the laboratory to enter clinical practice. Such advances have the potential to provide powerful tools that will improve health and fundamentally alter the practice of medicine.

Expectations are high that science will continue to yield great advances in the future, although the pace at which such discoveries will have a broad impact on people is unclear. The public has shown a willingness to support this important work, as evidenced by the growth in funding for the National Institutes of Health (NIH). Furthermore, concerns about bioterrorism and recurring and emerging infectious diseases will lead to more appeals for science to help alleviate and respond to such threats.

The trends described in Chapter 2 will also create a serious set of challenges for research in the coming decades. Not all advances will come from great breakthroughs. Health care also advances through a slow and steady series of incremental steps that refine knowledge and technology so that, cumulatively and over time, improvements in health result. There is a need for better knowledge of how to care most appropriately for and maintain the health of an aging and chronically ill population, and how to both improve the quality of care and contain its costs. Achieving progress in these areas will require improved understanding of the effectiveness of the clinical, organizational, and financial aspects of care so that safety, efficiency, and effectiveness can be designed into systems of care.

There is clear evidence of a gap in applying current knowledge in practice (Institute of Medicine, 2001b). Some patients are not receiving treatments that could be beneficial to them. According to one study, about 50 percent of patients for whom beta blocking agents were appropriate did not receive them (O'Connor et al., 1999). Some patients are receiving treatments that provide no benefit, or even cause harm. For example, calcium channel blocking agents were administered to 18 percent of patients with impaired left ventricular function, even though current guidelines recommend against their use in such cases (O'Connor et al., 1999). Likewise, over a 1-year period, 60 percent of Medicaid patients diagnosed with a cold filled a prescription for antibiotics (Shuster et al., 1996). Moreover, errors in clinical care result in death for thousands of people each year (Institute of

Medicine, 2000). Computer-based prescription order entry systems have been shown to reduce prescribing errors by one-half to three-quarters, but it is estimated that fewer than one-fifth of hospitals currently have such systems in place, and among those that do, fewer than 10 percent of orders are computerized (Doolan and Bates, 2002). In short, there is a large gap between what we know and what we do in terms of health care.

As noted in earlier chapters, unexplained variations in care have also been documented, suggesting the need for continued development of the evidence base. For example, among Medicare beneficiaries, overall discharge rates for medical conditions are 60 percent higher in Boston than in New Haven (Wennberg, 1999). Geographic analyses of Medicare beneficiaries have revealed that spending on health care in Miami was nearly 2.5 times that in Minneapolis (even after adjusting for age, sex, race, and price levels); visits to specialists in the last 6 months of life ranged from two times in Mason City, Iowa, to more than 25 times in Miami; and the proportion of eligible patients receiving beta blockers after a heart attack ranged from 5 to 92 percent (Wennberg et al., 2002). Variations in discharge rates, hospital days, and volume of outpatient visits among similar patients are found across age groups, in both inpatient and outpatient settings, for both acute and chronic conditions (Blumenthal, 1994; Ashton et al., 1999; Wennberg, 1999), and across different forms health insurance (Brook, 1997), and they persist even after controlling for differences in severity of illness. There is also growing recognition of how little is known about the effectiveness of many drugs, devices, practices, and procedures that are accepted as part of today's clinical practice (Garber, 1994), and of how difficult it is to synthesize across studies to advance knowledge.

Another concern is that the rising costs of care discussed in Chapter 2 are due in part to technological advancement itself. Technology affects the costs of health care by increasing the intensity of care provided to patients and by expanding the applications of the technology and the populations who can benefit (Neumann and Sandberg, 1998). At times, an innovation is introduced while its appropriate use remains uncertain, and is refined only after being applied in practice rather than before it has been diffused (Gelijns and Rosenberg, 1994). New technologies and increased use of existing technologies have been estimated to account for as much as two-thirds of the real annual increase in health spending (Blumenthal, 2001). Although technology may improve efficiency by reducing the cost of care per person, the number of eligible patients grows over time, so overall expenditures increase as well (Weisbrod and LaMay, 1999). Therefore, cost savings that may show up at the individual patient level are offset by overall higher expenditures due to increased use of the new technology (Gelijns and Rosenberg, 1994). A concern, then, is that increased investments in biomedical research will contribute excessively to rising health care costs

(Blumenthal, 2001) unless there is a better understanding of how to apply judiciously the innovations produced.

All of this suggests that, despite the great advances in knowledge achieved during the 20th century, much work remains to be done in the 21st century to develop a sound evidence base for health. An improved evidence base will result in part from basic research that will continue to uncover the fundamental mechanisms of disease and thereby reduce uncertainty in practice. For example, some complications from treatment or adverse reactions to medications may be reduced as a result of improvements in basic knowledge of treatment effects and patient responses. An improved evidence base will also result, however, from an increased emphasis on clinical, health services, and prevention research that will improve abilities to apply current knowledge, helping, for example, to eliminate recognized problems of overuse, underuse, and misuse (Chassin et al., 1998); assess the cost-efficient application of technology; or evaluate strategies designed to reduce health risks throughout the population. Thus AHCs need to participate in developing solutions to society's most pressing health problems not only by creating knowledge, but also by developing more systematic approaches for using research to encourage evidence-based patterns of practice, in order to improve health for both patients and populations.

WORKING ACROSS THE CONTINUUM OF RESEARCH

The translation of the discoveries of basic science into practice can be viewed as occurring along a continuum. This continuum has been defined in various ways, but generally progresses from basic research, to clinical research, to applied research—from fundamental science, through its application to patients, to studies of health and disease in populations (Frist, 2002; Association of American Medical Colleges, 1998). In addition, this committee considered the continuum in terms of the aim of the work—from discovery, to testing, to application, to evaluation. Discovery tends to rely on basic research; testing and application tend to rely on clinical research; and evaluation tends to rely on applied research. However, these distinctions are offered as a broad framework rather than a typology.

Basic biomedical research includes molecular biology, biochemistry, and cell biology and their application to mammalian, especially human, systems (Pober et al., 2001; Fontanarosa and DeAngelis, 2002). It often includes laboratory research using human material, such as cell cultures and DNA analyses (Oinonen et al., 2001). Advances in the fundamental sciences and the mechanisms of disease are critical to the development of diagnostic and therapeutic technologies and to the targeting of areas for subsequent clinical study (Gelijns and Thier, 2002).

Clinical research is defined by NIH as including three areas of study:

a) patient-oriented research, that is conducted with human subjects (or on material of human origin such as tissues, specimens, and cognitive phenomena) for which an investigator (or colleague) directly interacts with human subjects. This area of research includes mechanisms of human disease; therapeutic interventions; clinical trials; and development of new technologies; b) epidemiologic and behavioral studies; and c) outcomes research and health services research (National Institutes of Health, 1997, www.nih.gov/news/crp/97report/esecsum.htm#2define).

Although the above definition of clinical research includes aspects of study that relate to health services research, the committee has chosen to distinguish the latter from clinical research because it requires a distinct set of skills, focus, and expertise. Health services research is a multidisciplinary field of scientific investigation that studies how social factors, financing systems, organizational structures and processes, health technologies, and personal behaviors affect access to health care, the quality and cost of health care, and, ultimately, health and well-being. Its research domains are individuals, families, organizations, institutions, communities, and populations (AcademyHealth, 2002). It is often considered to also include research related to health policy and management.

Goldstein and Brown (1997) make an additional distinction between disease-oriented and patient-oriented research: the former is targeted toward understanding the pathogenesis or treatment of a disease but does not require direct contact with patients; the latter is performed by clinicians who observe, analyze, and manage individual patients. Disease-oriented research can be thought of as a bridge between basic and clinical research in that it focuses on a specific condition, as does clinical research, but it does not involve patient contact, as is the case with basic research. Goldstein and Brown perceive a rapid growth in disease-oriented research as compared with patient-oriented research for several reasons. First, technological breakthroughs in molecular biology attract scientifically oriented clinicians to basic science. Second, the pressures on the health care delivery system (combined with the rapid pace of research) make it difficult for any one person to be intensely involved in both types of research simultaneously. Third, basic research is often able to produce more clear-cut results as compared with patient-oriented research, making it easier to publish the results and obtain funding.

It is important to note that despite an implied order to the research process, the process by which a discovery is made, proven in practice, and diffused into the community is not necessarily linear (Gelijns and Rosenberg, 1994). For example, an innovation that enters practice usually undergoes a continuing process of refinement and development after its introduction.

Moreover, an experience in the clinical setting may feed back into the laboratory, leading to the development of additional fundamental knowledge about a condition; that is, the order of the process as outlined above may be reversed. The stages of the continuum also tend to occur in a discrete and often unrelated fashion. For example, the cost-effectiveness of a discovery is usually assessed separately from its clinical effectiveness, typically after it has been introduced into a clinical setting.

Furthermore, although the continuum described above encompasses different types of research, they are all interrelated. Basic research rarely produces findings in the laboratory that can be used immediately in clinical practice. One means of translating basic research into practice is through clinical trials, but they leave many unanswered questions as well. For example, clinical trials generally do not consider impacts on overall treatment patterns for affected or multiple populations and rarely examine the costs or cost-effectiveness of an intervention (that is, they focus on efficacy more than effectiveness). Even after testing for clinical safety and effectiveness, questions remain about how to integrate the improvements into everyday practice for the average patient. Health services, outcomes, effectiveness, and other evaluative research can complement the work done in biomedical and clinical research by addressing such issues as how to organize and finance care, how to measure and evaluate its quality, how to involve patients in their care, how to encourage patients to adopt behaviors that promote health and prevent disease, and how to facilitate the adoption of scientific knowledge (Horwitz, 2002).

Additionally, although the various forms of research are interrelated, they are typically conducted by different scientists and funded separately. Increased coordination and collaboration will be required to meet growing demands for rapid improvements in health care and for a greater focus on the types of research that answer questions about what does and does not work (Stryer et al., 2000). This is not to suggest that research is useful only if it has an immediate impact, but rather that the ultimate goal is to produce knowledge that can help people.

AHCs have been shaped by basic research, dating back to a 1945 report by Vannevar Bush that established a system for federal support of research conducted primarily by independent investigators, based in universities, and awarded funds through a process of peer review (Association of American Medical Colleges, 1998). During the 1950s and 1960s, NIH believed that diseases would be cured when science provided an understanding of their physiology; the result was significant growth in the basic science departments of medical schools (Goldstein and Brown, 1997). Basic science is viewed as flourishing today because of growth in NIH funding levels for this work and in the number of basic researchers (Goldstein and Brown, 1997).

Although almost all AHCs receive funding from NIH, this funding is concentrated in a subset of these institutions. It is estimated that in 2000, approximately one-third of NIH funding to AHCs went to the top 10 institutions (mainly to the medical schools), which received an average of about $280 million each; the next 40 institutions received about 50 percent of the money, for an average about $110 million each; and the remaining institutions received about 15 percent of the total (Anderson, 2002). Between 1987 and 1997, the proportion of NIH research awards to the 10 most research-intensive institutions increased, while those to the less-intensive institutions decreased (Moy et al., 2000). The reliance on NIH funding could create financial constraints on AHCs' ability to maintain current levels of basic research. Sustaining the recent rate of growth in the NIH budget would require 14 to 16 percent annual increases; increases of less than 6 percent would squeeze current funding levels. The president's budget for 2004–2007 includes an annual growth in funding for NIH of around 2 percent (Korn, 2002).

AHCs have also been affected by a shift in the way clinical trials are conducted. The volume of clinical trials is growing rapidly, and the trials are also becoming dispersed to many sites. Private companies, known as contract research organizations (CROs), manage clinical trials for pharmaceutical companies. CROs are one mechanism for expanding the capacity to conduct trials, and they also allow physicians in the community to become involved in clinical research. At the same time, however, more clinical trials are now being conducted outside of AHCs than within them. It has been estimated that investigators in AHCs represent about 46 percent of all those involved in research, down from 80 percent a decade earlier, with the majority of industry funding for clinical trials being allocated to community-based efforts (Morin et al., 2002). The market for CROs is estimated to grow by approximately 15 to 20 percent per year, leading them to dominate the market for clinical trials research (Rettig, 2000).

Obstacles to Conducting Research Across the Continuum

AHCs need to consider how they can participate in research across the full continuum described above. Despite growing interest in measuring the effectiveness of medical interventions and developing more valid and robust indictors of effectiveness, AHCs face a number of obstacles in accomplishing these objectives. Several such obstacles are considered here, including training of clinical investigators, creation of the organizational processes required for research across the continuum, inadequate federal funding levels, and ethical issues.

Training of Clinical Investigators

A major obstacle to conducting research across the continuum is the supply of clinical researchers. Whereas the number of basic researchers is growing, clinical advances are threatened by a lack of growth in the numbers of clinical investigators (Goldstein and Brown, 1997). It is estimated that only about 11 percent of medical school graduates plan a career devoted exclusively or significantly to research (Nathan, 2002). A study by the National Research Council (2000) revealed that the number of Ph.D.'s awarded in the basic biomedical sciences is well above that needed; however, there is evidence of a decline in the number of physicians conducting research. Unfortunately, data for determining such trends are highly limited as no objective data source exists (Crowley and Thier, 1996; National Research Council, 2000).

There are several barriers to pursuing a career in clinical research. Clinical researchers obtain training in both biomedical sciences and clinical practice, both of which are increasing in complexity. Major debts are incurred from the many years of training required to acquire expertise in both research methods and clinical care, and the demands of retaining skills in both areas over time are enormous (Crowley and Thier, 1996; Nathan, 2002). The pressure to pay their debts causes investigators to spend more time in clinical care than in research (Wolf, 2002). Furthermore, there are fewer training opportunities in clinical, health services, and prevention research than in laboratory research in that the latter appears to be favored by both funding agencies (particularly NIH) and AHCs themselves (Crowley and Thier, 1996; Wolf, 2002). A lack of predictable support also raises concern about the ability to raise sufficient funds to conduct the research. This concern is particularly acute for clinical investigators who train until their mid-thirties and then may be unable to raise sufficient funds to pursue their intended work (Wolf, 2002). A lack of core institutional resources is also seen as a barrier, particularly for health services research centers (Nathan, 2002; Kindig et al., 1999).

In recent years, NIH has attempted to address these concerns by creating a series of awards for new and midcareer investigators involved in clinical research, as well as educational loan repayment programs (Wolf, 2002). The expansion of training opportunities at NIH-supported General Clinical Research Centers may be another approach to increase support for clinical researchers (Vaitukaitis, 2000). These centers receive support for research infrastructure, including specialized staff and computer systems, and many are located at AHCs.

Clinical training programs should ensure better exposure to quality research experiences to encourage more clinicians to consider careers in research. Students exposed to research during their clinical training may be more likely to engage in research activities later in their career (Kalfoglou and Sung, 2002; Institute of Medicine, 1994). Even those students not choosing a research career can gain an understanding of scientific methods and the capabilities needed for critically evaluating the research literature (Institute of Medicine, 1994). If students are expected to read the research literature and understand the latest findings surrounding the new sciences, they need to learn the language of the field. These are regarded as valuable skills even for those who do not conduct research directly (Kalfoglou and Sung, 2002).

Creation of Organizational Processes

Clinical and health services research tends to be organized differently from basic science research. Basic biomedical research is typically carried out by an individual investigator or team of investigators from the same field. In contrast, the power of translational research derives from its combination with basic and population sciences; more interdisciplinary approaches are required, as well as better integration of medical, health, social, and behavioral sciences and other areas of the life sciences. The emphasis on research performed by individual scientists may have worked well in the past but is "not a prescription for success in clinical research" (Nathan, 2002, p. 2426). Some believe that the individual investigator who tries to do it all will flounder (Nathan, 2002), given that the necessary expertise will reside in a team of researchers rather than an individual, as is becoming increasingly true for many types of research.

The interdisciplinary approaches that are central to translating research into practice are not well rewarded either by external funders or within the AHC structure. Research studies on patients appear to be held in low esteem by NIH study sections (Nathan, 2002). Within AHCs, investigators engaged in patient- and population-based studies have not been promoted as rapidly as individual scientists conducting basic research and have more difficulty in obtaining discretionary resources (The Commonwealth Fund Task Force on Academic Health Centers, 2000). In evaluating individuals for promotion, AHCs have typically emphasized NIH grants to individual investigators as well as the ability to publish in leading journals, which is facilitated by having received an NIH grant. Moreover, institutional support within AHCs is allocated through individual departments (Pober et al., 2001; Kindig et al., 1999; Nathan, 2002). Thus, individual excellence is emphasized, rather than the collaborative efforts required.

The organization of AHCs by academic department is designed to facilitate interactions among researchers within the same discipline. Translational research may require the aggregation of expertise across a very diverse set of disciplines, both health and nonhealth related. For example, the evidence-based practice centers funded by the Agency for Healthcare Research and Quality comprise teams with highly diverse expertise and skill sets (Agency for Healthcare Research and Quality, 2002). Organizational boundaries may be crossed not only within the medical school, for example, but also throughout the AHC and even across the university, tapping expertise from economics, engineering, mathematics, psychology, and so on.

In one example at an AHC, Dartmouth University created the Center for Evaluative Clinical Sciences in 1989 as a locus for scientists and clinical scholars from across the university who conduct research on issues related to measuring, organizing, and improving the health care system (Center for Evaluative Clinical Sciences, 2003). The center gathers physicians, epidemiologists, psychologists, sociologists, economists, medical geographers, statisticians, and others to answer such questions as how well medical and surgical procedures actually work, how health care resources are distributed and used, how patients value medical interventions and their consequences, and how the quality of medical and surgical care can be continuously improved. In another example, the University of Virginia created a Department of Health Evaluation Sciences in 1995 to provide multidisciplinary scientific and analytical services to its Health Sciences Center and the rest of the university. These services involve examining the development of new approaches and strategies in such areas as the prognosis and clinical and genetic risk assessment of health and disease; medical decision making; and medical practice delivery for individuals and populations (University of Virginia Health System, 2003).

Another organizational issue is how oversight of research is performed, which may not match the way research is conducted. Institutional review boards (IRBs) were established in the 1960s (Moses and Martin, 2001). Since then, however, studies have increasingly involved multiple institutions and settings. If a study seeks to examine the clinical and cost outcomes of care for a group of patients undergoing a cardiac procedure in a hospital, that study is reviewed by the hospital's IRB. However, if the researchers want to understand outcomes beyond the hospital stay, for example, by examining care at a rehabilitative unit and at the outpatient clinic, the study may encounter separate IRBs for each care setting, even within the same system (Barbara McNeil, personal communication, 2002). The problem is multiplied for multi-institutional studies. These processes add both time and cost to the research effort. IRB processes must be redesigned to ensure adequate protection for study participants in order to gain their trust and participation, without placing an excessive burden on investigators. Since clinical and often health services research involves patients, the pressure to address this issue will grow.

Finally, a lack of good information systems is another type of organizational obstacle. As discussed previously, translational research in the 21st century will depend on access to good information systems (Manning, 2000). Research in biomedical fields such as genomics generates immense amounts of data to be analyzed. Correlation of genotypes with phenotypes will require access to longitudinal clinical information and large numbers of patients. Additionally, measuring the effectiveness of interventions and assessing in both clinical and cost terms their impacts on practice patterns and outcomes often requires overlaying data collection on clinical practice. And enhanced surveillance of disease outbreaks or bioterrorism events will require improved information systems that can link the acute care and public health systems. Such data collection needs to be integrated into care processes and other routine procedures, or the data become too difficult to collect and/or too expensive to harvest. Most studies on effectiveness and outcomes have relied on administrative data for the conduct of retrospective analyses; however, if clinical and health services research is to affect health care policies, practices, and outcomes, more timely data, including real-time data, will be needed (Stryer et al., 2000). To this end, there is a crucial need for better information and communications systems with capabilities for knowledge management and decision support.

Inadequate Federal Funding of Clinical and Health Services Research

Support for research comes from a variety of sources. The bulk of federal funding for health-related research is provided to and by NIH. Funding for NIH grew from $3 billion in 1980 to more than $20 billion in 2001 (U.S. General Accounting Office, 2001), fueling the growth in basic science since, as noted, the majority of funds has been allocated to laboratory-based biomedical research (Schroeder et al., 1989). In 2001, NIH awarded about $16 billion in extramural research awards, about half of which went to AHCs (National Institutes of Health, 2002a). Health-related research support is also provided by the Veterans Health Administration, the Agency for Healthcare Research and Quality, the Centers for Disease Control and Prevention, the Department of Defense, the Centers for Medicare and Medicaid Services, the Indian Health Service, the Department of Energy, the Environmental Protection Agency, and even the National Aeronautics and Space Administration (National Science and Technology Council, 2000).

Estimates of support for basic biomedical, clinical, and health services research vary. In estimating the proportion of NIH support for clinical research, the NIH Director's Panel on Clinical Research used a very broad definition of clinical research that included mechanisms of human disease, therapeutic interventions, clinical trials, development of new technologies, epidemiologic and behavioral studies, and outcomes and health services research (National Institutes of Health, 1997). At that time, the panel estimated that 38 percent of the NIH budget was devoted to clinical research. Some believe, however, that this figure overestimates the resources devoted to clinical studies in that some studies may contribute to understanding of disease without directly involving humans (Schechter, 1998). Other estimates suggest that a lower proportion of NIH funding is devoted to clinical research. For example, an earlier analysis by the Institute of Medicine (1994) revealed that 90 percent of NIH extramural grants supported basic science research and only 10 percent clinical research (Institute of Medicine, 1994).

Federal support for clinical and health services research has not been at a level comparable to that devoted to basic biomedical research (Sung et al., 2003). In fiscal year 2000, the total research budget was approximately $21 billion for NIH, the Department of Defense, the Centers for Disease Control and Prevention, the Department of Energy, the Department of Veterans Affairs, the Health Resources and Services Administration, the Agency for Healthcare Research and Quality, the Food and Drug Administration, and the Centers for Medicare and Medicaid Services combined. The budget for clinical research was estimated at approximately $7 billion, plus an additional estimated $1.3 billion dedicated to outcomes and health services research. Funding for health research aimed at populations and community-based prevention is low, and not a priority in government funding or academia (Institute of Medicine, 2002e).

Support for health research is also provided by private industry. Health-related research and development by private industry increased 382 percent between 1985 and 1997 (The Commonwealth Fund Task Force on Academic Health Centers, 1999). Domestic research and development expenditures by members of the Pharmaceutical Research and Manufacturers of America (2002) were estimated to total almost $24 billion in 2001. Investment in research by the top 20 pharmaceutical companies has more than doubled in recent years (Morin et al., 2002). AHCs have benefited from this investment by forging partnerships with private industry to conduct complex studies and enable each sector to tap the expertise and resources of the other. Health-related research is also conducted by other schools and departments of a university, as well as by independent research institutions, consulting firms, managed care plans, hospitals, professional societies, foundations, and government agencies (Kindig et al., 1999).

It is difficult to obtain precise figures on patterns of overall spending for different types of health-related research. Part of the difficulty is due to definitional overlaps, as noted previously. In addition, however, there is no explicit policy toward shaping research and development in health care (Weisbrod and LaMay, 1999); thus there is no frame of reference, making it difficult to array data consistently across agencies and funders. The development of a well-formulated research agenda for basic, clinical, health services, and prevention research could permit the identification of priorities based on good measurement, better public dialogue between policy makers and the users of research on how to incorporate scientific advances into practice and policy, and improved collaboration across the many parties that are interested in and benefit from such research (Frist, 2002).

Ethical Issues Related to Research

New areas of research generate new ethical issues of serious concern. We discuss here only some of the ethical concerns that must be addressed.

First, although both AHCs and private industry can bring benefits to research partnerships, issues related to conflicts of interest can arise, including financial conflicts of interest, potential biases in reporting positive results, researchers' access to complete data, and effects on research priorities (Korn, 2000; Gelijns and Thier, 2002; U.S. General Accounting Office, 2001). Furthermore, it has been suggested that evaluative research requires some distance in the relationship between the developer of a product or device and its evaluator (Gelijns and Thier, 2002). Therefore, there is a potential conflict of interest for AHCs if they are engaged as both the developer and evaluator of new technology. Some AHCs are establishing separate research institutes to facilitate collaborations and reduce conflicts of interest by housing the research outside of the AHC (Moses and Martin, 2001). In general, AHC and industry relationships should be formed with recognition of the potential for conflicts of interest at both the individual and the organizational levels, and with attention to the expectations each party brings to the work and obligations for disclosure (Broder, 2002; Institute of Medicine, 2001, 2002b).

Serious ethical concerns also arise from emerging technologies in genetics, stem cell research, and cloning, affecting work across the research continuum. Ensuring the confidentiality of patient information while making it accessible to researchers can be expected to require continuing policy attention. As studies on humans become more complex, concerns also arise regarding how patients can be protected and adequately informed of the risks associated with the research in which they participate (Institute of Medicine, 2001, 2002).

The committee also notes the importance of other ethical issues, such as confidentiality of data, conflicts over tissue sampling, and the uniqueness and special handling of genetic data. These issues merit additional study but were beyond the scope of this committee's charge.

IMPLICATIONS FOR THE FUTURE

Society needs the results of work done across the entire research continuum. Basic research will continue to be important to produce the fundamental knowledge and tools needed to improve health. However, clinical, health services, and prevention research will also be necessary to improve understanding of how to improve health and to translate the findings of basic research into clinical and community settings so its benefits will reach people.

In the coming decades, AHCs will need to increase their emphasis on research across the continuum, including clinical, health services, and prevention research in addition to basic research. All such work needs to be recognized, rewarded, and supported. Meeting this need will not require that each AHC expand its research portfolio. One way to encourage greater emphasis across the continuum is through collaboration (Goldstein and Brown, 1997). The individual clinician–researcher represents one model, but another approach is clinicians and researchers working together. Collaborations are being created organizationally through large research institutes and centers, but even a few individuals working together can generate important advances. For example, the discovery of the anti-inflammatory properties of cortisone was the product of collaboration among a clinician, a chemist, and a pharmaceutical company (Goldstein and Brown, 1997). As noted earlier, such collaborations, especially across disciplines, are not adequately rewarded in AHCs, which emphasize individual achievement.

Funding agencies also need to support and foster collaborations across the research continuum. At present, it is difficult for agencies to support interdisciplinary approaches, either by funding research led by an interdisciplinary team or by providing interagency funding. Furthermore, the interrelated fields of information technology, biological sciences, and materials sciences may offer some of the most promising research in the future (Frist, 2002) but are not generally linked together by the various funding agencies to maximize their potential. Federal agencies need to improve their coordination in support of both research and research training programs, and to support much-needed collaborations across researchers and institutions.

CHAPTER 6

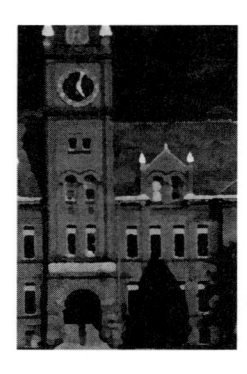

THE CONSEQUENCES OF CURRENT FINANCING METHODS FOR THE FUTURE ROLES OF AHCS

The previous chapters have laid out an approach for how AHCs should adapt their roles to meet the public's needs in the 21st century. Although many responsibilities for accomplishing this fall to the leadership of the AHCs, financing policies should facilitate and reward those AHCs that undertake the transformation asked for in this report.

AHCs are currently financed through a variety of sources that vary for each role. The academic functions of education and research are particularly dependent on public financing, whereas the patient care role is supported through a combination of public and private funding. For most AHCs, the education and research roles are not believed to be self-supporting but are subsidized from revenues derived from patient care. As patient care revenues have become constrained due to changes by both public and private payers, the funds available to subsidize these other activities are also constrained.

This chapter reviews the current financing of education, research, and clinical care in AHCs; identifies behaviors brought about by current financing methods; projects the consequences of continuing current financing methods; and identifies policy options that might harmonize the apparent discrepancy between society's future needs and current financing methods. The focus of this discussion is on AHCs' roles, not on the AHCs themselves. An assumption underlying the analysis in this chapter is that, regardless of mission, financial incentives affect behavior. Thus, depending on how financing trends evolve, the manner in which the roles are funded and organized could differ markedly from today's status quo.

The committee finds the following:

- Current approaches for financing the roles of AHCs will not support the future directions in which the roles need to develop to meet the public's needs.
- AHCs are heavily dependent upon public sources of funding, which are likely face problems in sustaining their levels of support in the future due to noncontrollable demographic shifts that affect program revenues and demands, especially in Medicare.
- Policy makers will be faced with very difficult decisions if they are to ensure adequate levels of support for activities carried out by AHCs. But AHCs themselves will have to make hard decisions about what can be done within the level of resources available.
- The prior chapters in this report have laid out an aggressive agenda for change *and innovation*. Financing for the AHCs' roles needs to support the process of change that is being asked of AHCs. In some cases, it may be possible to make adjustments within current methods; in other cases, more fundamental changes may be required.

CURRENT STATUS OF FINANCING CLINICAL EDUCATION, RESEARCH, AND PATIENT CARE IN AHCS

AHCs receive financial support for their roles from a variety of sources. The funding sources vary for each role. These funding patterns are only briefly reviewed here as they have been covered in great detail by other groups. Those interested in more extended discussions of the specific formulas for current payment methods should obtain reports produced other groups, such as The Commonwealth Task Force on Academic Health Centers, the Council on Graduate Medical Education, or the Medicare Payment Advisory Commission.

Support for clinical education is supported through a combination of cross-subsidies from patient care revenues and explicit funding, primarily from public sources, particularly for medical residents. Medicare pays hospitals for its share of residents' stipends, faculty salaries, and related expenses (called direct graduate medical education, or DGME, payments) plus an add-on to their inpatient diagnosis-related group (DRG) rates based on the number of residents per bed (called indirect medical education, or IME, payments). In 2000, Medicare provided almost $6 billion in IME payments, about $2 billion in DGME payments, and about $260 million for nursing and allied health programs (Boyle and Fisher, 2002; Medicare Payment Advisory Commission, 2001).

Additional support for health professions training is provided by the Health Resources and Services Administration (HRSA) Bureau of Health Professions (about $400 million in 2002) and to individual scientists by the National Institutes of Health (about $650 million in 2002) (National Institutes of Health, 2003). State Medicaid programs, non-Medicaid state appropriations, Veterans Administration, and Department of Defense also contribute public dollars to financing clinical education. While some of these dollars are devoted to non-physician training, by far the majority funds physician education. Medicare currently pays AHCs an average of approximately $65,000 per resident per year (Appendix A).

The principal source of research dollars flowing to AHCs is the National Institutes of Health (NIH). AHCs received an average per institution in excess of $60 million in NIH funds in 2000, over $60,000 per faculty member (appendix A). The amount received per institution was somewhat variable, with the top 50 NIH recipients getting well in excess of $100 million and over $100,000 per faculty member (Appendix A). Total federal spending for biomedical research has been estimated at approximately $25 billion in 2000, with private foundation support contributing approximately $8 billion to $10 billion, and private industry contributing as much as $55 billion to $60 billion (although only a fraction of the latter goes to AHCs) (Moses and Martin, 2001). While the budget of the NIH has increased rapidly over the past several years, the research expenditures by private organizations has increased even more rapidly such that the proportion of biomedical research financed by industry has been increasing. For AHCs, however, the NIH remains the principal funding source for their research enterprises. Over the 1990–2000 period, the amount of NIH funding per AHC increased an average of 126 percent (Appendix A).

AHCs do not differ markedly from other institutions in patient care revenue sources. Roughly, 30 percent of revenues come from Medicare, 20 percent from Medicaid, and the remainder primarily from private insurance. AHCs do differ, however, in their extent of uncompensated care, primarily for care to the poor. In 2000, uncompensated care was about 7 percent of their costs,[1] about 3 percentage points higher than other large, urban nonteaching hospitals (Dobson et al., 2002). In part to compensate hospitals that serve a disproportionate share of the poor, Medicare and Medicaid pay a supplement to inpatient rates called the disproportionate share (DSH) adjustment. The Medicare adjustment, which is based on proportions of patients who are Medicaid and who are combined Medicare-Medicaid, is by far the larger of the two. In 2000, AHCs received an

---

[1]Defined as the sum of bad debt and charity care charges converted to costs by a hospital-specific ratio of costs to charges, minus the tax allowances for bad debt and charity care.

average of about $1500 per Medicare discharge in DSH supplemental payments (Appendix A).

It is important to recognize that most of the dollars flowing into AHCs are fungible; that is, they can be used for a variety of purposes regardless of the reasons they were paid (except for research grant dollars). GME and DSH dollars flow to the hospital's general operating revenues. Patient-care revenues obtained by AHC hospitals and faculty practice plans have historically been deployed both to cover necessary expenses and to finance discretionary spending related to institutional activities. Thus, the extent of support for education and research within an AHC is a function of external funding but is greatly affected by internal decisions about how funds are to be used (Kirch, 2002).

OBSERVATIONS REGARDING CURRENT FINANCING METHODS AND AMOUNTS

A number of general observations can be made about current support for the financing of the AHC roles.

First, the financing of clinical education is Medicare-dependent. The sum of IME and DGME payments to AHCs far exceeds support for clinical education from other sources. As such, AHCs are dependent on a flow of Medicare inpatients to generate GME revenues. In particular, IME payments are calculated as an add-on to Medicare inpatient DRG rates to compensate hospitals for the costs of patient care (for Medicare patients) associated with operating approved physician training programs, although evidence finds that the IME add-on exceeds the "empirical level" at which the costs of caring for Medicare patients in teaching hospitals exceed costs in nonteaching institutions of treating clinically similar patients (MedPAC, 2002; COGME, 2000).

The private sector has also become less willing to subsidize education costs in its patient care payments to hospitals, in part, due to the growth of managed care in recent years and pressures to contain the costs of care. In the past, private payers routinely paid premiums to teaching hospitals on the order of 25 percent more than what would be paid for similar services in community hospitals. Now, according to some reports, managed care organizations are negotiating agreements with teaching hospitals with premiums no greater than 5 to 10 percent in order for the hospital to be included on a preferred provider list (Anderson et al., 1999; Committee on the Roles of Academic Health Centers in the 21st Century, 2002).

Second, the public subsidy of graduate medical education is being questioned. Historically, the achievement of a well-trained physician workforce has been seen as a justification for public subsidy of graduate medical education (Anderson et al., 2001; The Commonwealth Fund Task Force on

Academic Health Centers, 1997a). Today, this "public good" rationale is not universally accepted (Newhouse and Wilensky, 2001; Gbadebo and Reinhardt, 2001). The fact that economists do not believe that medical education meets the textbook definition of a public good is probably less important than public dissatisfaction with the amount and distribution of these payments. The current financing method has encouraged teaching hospitals to employ more residents and arguably has contributed to physician oversupply, maldistribution, and specialty imbalance (Young and Coffman, 1998; Institute of Medicine, 1996). For example, the inability of the graduate medical education system to produce more specialists in geriatric medicine in the face of obvious demographic trends has caused some observers to question whether the public subsidy provides incentives to meet public needs.

The amount of Medicare payments has varied enormously among hospitals in ways that are hard to relate to public objectives. Most importantly, the payment system does not permit any accountability for achievement of public goals regarding the size, composition, and location of the physician workforce, nor does it permit balancing subsidies to promote availability of nonphysician health care workers (Salsberg, 2001). Consequently, the DGME and IME adjustments are targets for cuts in the annual federal budget cycle (Matherlee, 2001). While cuts have not been implemented in every budget bill, the trend is clearly in the direction of reducing Medicare subsidy of physician education and is likely to remain so for the foreseeable future.

Third, the financing of clinical education is mismatched with public needs. The current financing of clinical education that is so heavily reliant on Medicare DGME and IME payments is also oriented toward hospital inpatient and acute care and is primarily physician oriented. In contrast, the population medical needs, abetted both by demographic and medical technology trends, is moving in the direction of home and community care (for living with chronic illness) and is being met through increasingly sophisticated services provided in outpatient and office-based settings. The population is not only aging but is also becoming more racially and culturally diverse. Training in interdisciplinary approaches to treatment, especially preferred for treating chronic illness and senior health problems, is not encouraged by the present financing system for education.

To be sure, some changes in financing orientation have been made in recent years. Some funds have been made available to subsidize nursing education and, given the present shortage, more help is likely to be on the way. The DGME and IME payments have been structured so as not to discourage hospitals from deploying their residents in community settings, to encourage primary care residency training, and the number of residents qualifying for subsidy payments has been capped (Matherlee, 2001). These changes are slight, however, in relation to the totality of the inpatient-based Medicare subsidy and the changing nature of society's needs.

Fourth, the research role shares some of the stresses experienced by medical education. While research in AHCs is funded quite differently from clinical education, some of the threats to funding continuation appear similar. Historically, for example, growth in both the education and research enterprises in AHCs was accepted as economically beneficial (Blumenthal and Meyer, 1996). Today, AHCs face continued incentives to grow these enterprises with no assurance that the added costs will be covered by direct payments or by surplus clinical revenues (Matherlee, 1995). This is in part due to the reduced willingness of private payers to subsidize the costs of both education and research.

Research funding through the National Institutes of Health has grown substantially in recent years, but so has competition for NIH dollars. In addition, research funding by private organizations has grown as a proportion of the total, outpacing the increase in NIH funding. The mechanisms through which the public interest is served by these increases is a hodgepodge of disease advocacy, profit seeking, and investigator-initiated pursuit of discoveries in basic research. Although the public support for research subsidy remains strong, it is unlikely that the NIH budget will continue to increase at its recent pace (Korn, 2002), and the shift in funding toward the private sector implies a greater orientation toward discoveries and inventions with commercial potential (Matherlee, 2000; Moses and Martin, 2001).

Fifth, the role of AHCs in translational and applied research is not supported by current financing methods. A number of organizations and individuals have advocated in favor of research institutions becoming more involved in research that converts basic discoveries into cost-effective medical interventions (Institute of Medicine, 2002; Nathan, 1998). The "model" of basic research investigators competing for new and continuation grants from the NIH is not entirely compatible, however, with AHCs becoming more involved in clinical, health services and prevention research. The sources of clinical research funds (predominantly private), the methods of competing for research funding, and the disciplines required to conduct such research, are very different. Funding for research that does have a translational orientation, such as grants from the Agency for Healthcare Research and Quality (AHRQ), is minuscule compared to the levels of funding from NIH. Moreover, the costs associated with "vetting" new technologies before they diffuse into mainstream clinical practice are seldom supported by research funding or recognized by payment systems.

Sixth, surplus revenues from clinical services in AHCs are shrinking. As noted above, private payers' willingness to subsidize non-patient-care costs in AHCs is diminishing as pressure is placed on private health plans to control spending. Private payers are looking elsewhere for routine services and seeking arrangements with "centers of excellence" for specialized services. Pressure is also exerted on Medicare and state Medicaid programs to control the growth of program spending. At the same time, medical technology advances are pushing services into the outpatient setting where (at least for Medicare) operating margins are smaller than for inpatient services. As a result of these trends, surplus funds available in AHCs to subsidize their roles are shrinking and are likely to shrink further.

Seventh, the AHC safety net role is being stretched. Many of the costs of caring for the uninsured poor are borne by AHCs and other safety net hospitals. GME and DSH payments help to defray these costs, but they are not well targeted. Medicare DSH payments, for example, are based on the hospital's Medicaid caseload. This mechanism creates an incentive for hospitals to accept Medicaid inpatients (since these patients will increase the add-on to Medicare inpatient payments) but a disincentive to accept patients with no insurance. In addition, hospitals in states with relatively generous Medicaid eligibility requirements have higher DSH payments and less uncompensated care, other things being equal, whereas hospitals in states with stringent Medicaid eligibility have lower DSH payments but more uncompensated care (The Commonwealth Fund Task Force on Academic Health Centers, 1997b). Thus DSH payments are not well targeted to cover the costs of uncompensated care to the uninsured poor. The methodology also encourages the provision of hospital services rather than the development of care models that can better meet the needs of this population.

The persistence of the large segment of uninsured population in the U.S. combined with pressure on state budgets to control spending suggest that the problem of uncompensated care is unlikely to dissipate. The increased unwillingness of private payers to voluntarily subsidize higher costs in AHCs also contributes to the problem. The public relies on some AHCs and other hospitals to provide safety net services to the uninsured poor. Except for the relatively few public hospitals whose budgets are funded by state and local governments, there are few payment mechanisms to directly compensate most hospitals for the costs of this public service.

FUTURE CONSEQUENCES OF CONTINUING CURRENT FINANCING METHODS

This section assesses the consequences of a "straight-line" continuation of current financing methods in light of trends in population needs, technology advancement, and cost pressures discussed earlier in this report. The future contemplated here is sufficiently distant that it is beyond effective consideration by our current policy decision-making apparatus, but sufficiently near that prudent organizations would incorporate consideration of it into long-range planning. The discussion begins with alternative scenarios describing the future of public and private health care financing, and continues with possible consequences for the AHC roles.

In terms of public financing for health care, health care spending as a proportion of Gross Domestic Product (GDP) will continue to increase, with the result that the future federal policy environment is likely to be dominated by the need to limit the growth of Medicare spending. The leading edge of the population segment known as the "baby boomers" (people born between 1946 and 1964) will begin to age into Medicare eligibility in 2011. The effect on Medicare spending will be slight at first (most of the young baby-boomer seniors will be relatively healthy), but eventually the health problems of this population segment, combined with its sheer size, will have a profound effect on Medicare spending. Under current law, Medicare spending is projected to double from historical levels to 4.5 percent of GDP in 2030, about the time that the Medicare Health Insurance trust fund is projected to become insolvent (Social Security Administration and Medicare Boards of Trustees, 2002). The potential consequences of this trend for taxes, the national debt, and/or the "crowding out" effect on nonentitlement spending will place enormous pressure on the federal government to limit Medicare spending.

These possible consequences could have mixed effects on health care provider organizations. On one hand, there is likely to be substantial money in the system as the proportion of GDP devoted to health care continues to grow. On the other hand, providers who rely on Medicare and other federal programs for funding are likely to be affected by efforts to control federal spending. Of course, many developments on the national policy scene could affect this scenario. Efforts to restructure Medicare, such as proposals contemplated by the National Bipartisan Commission on the Future of Medicare in 1999, may be resurrected and implemented. It is also possible that a national system of health financing, such as that advanced in the first Clinton term, could be enacted. While such changes would alter the picture considerably, the failure of the federal government to create such reforms in the past suggests the likelihood of their being enacted in the near future as unlikely.

In the private sector, efforts to control health care spending increases will likely create a new breed of informed consumers with financial incentives to purchase cost-effective products and services. As noted earlier in this report, a number of trends appear to be leading to consumers of the future having more direct responsibility for their health care purchases. On one hand, the explosion in medical technology advances is creating new diagnostic and treatment options. Direct-to-consumer advertising and the Internet will continue to provide consumers opportunities to be informed (and sometimes misinformed) about the strengths and weaknesses of the options before them. On the other hand, the introduction of new forms of cost-sharing in insured plans, combined with the persistence of a large segment of the population which is uninsured or underinsured, suggests that consumers will have a direct financial incentive to seek alternatives that minimize out-of-pocket costs. Cost pressures facing payers are likely to result in expansions of such concepts as three-tiered drug copayments and preferred provider arrangements that contain costs by shifting part of the responsibility to consumers. As noted before, the same concept is being applied to hospitals in some areas.

As in the case of the governmental programs, the future presents the potential for mixed consequences for providers. More money will flow into the system as new technologies are brought on line and consumers continue to demand all that technology has to offer. In addition, it is at least possible that some of these new technologies will be cost-decreasing. Also, reforms in the tort system may alter how health plans make coverage decisions if it is possible to substitute clinically equivalent but less costly alternatives without threat of malpractice proceedings and awards. Despite these possibilities, it still seems likely that the consumer of the future will seek to have their perceived health needs met in settings and by providers where their out-of-pocket costs are minimized.

A continuation of current methods of financing, in light of future trends, presents difficulties for AHCs to continue to fulfill clinical education, research, and patient care roles as they presently do. Many of the trends affecting health care financing in the future are well under way. In every case, the stresses experienced by AHCs in the face of such trends are likely to intensify in the absence of financing change.

In the case of clinical education, a continuation of current financing methods will exacerbate the growing imbalance between the acute, inpatient, physician orientation of financing and the chronic, outpatient, multidisciplinary nature of patient needs. Continued variability in GME payments, coupled with the lack of accountability to public health care workforce goals, will continue to undermine the public-good rationale for Medicare subsidy of medical education costs. Eventually, these subsidies may fall to a point where hiring residents will appear financially unattractive to many AHCs.

In the case of research, a slowdown in growth of NIH and other publicly funded research, coupled with shrinking patient care surpluses, will exacerbate the problem of unreimbursed overhead costs. Much new research, especially that funded within the private sector, will be conducted outside of AHCs in settings consistent with trends toward outpatient care for chronic illness. AHCs may be faced with incentives to downsize their research enterprises, set clearer priorities, and/or seek new commercial development opportunities.

In the case of patient care, the ability of many AHCs to generate excess revenues to support mission activities will diminish and possibly disappear altogether. Safety net institutions, in particular, will be under extreme pressure to continue to provide uncompensated care to the uninsured poor. The ratio of routine to specialized services will likely lessen as payers will seek less expensive services in alternative settings. AHCs are likely to respond by seeking new opportunities to leverage their role as developers of new technology into enhanced revenues by demanding payment for their most unique services, in essence, exploiting their monopoly niche in the subset of specialized services that are uniquely provided by AHCs. However, as the patient care setting becomes more specialized, the patient mix is less representative of the general population, potentially affecting the education role.

POLICY OPTIONS

What financing policy options might be pursued to reshape the education, research, and patient care roles and ensure that they are fulfilled?[2] Below we examine options for changing financing in each of the three areas. *Incremental* changes are those that can be accomplished with current financing structures remaining in place. *Fundamental* changes are those that would discard the current structures and replace them with new financing structures. In some cases the discussion below refers to specific changes in federal financing policy; in others it refers to actions that AHCs may take in response to a changing financing environment.

Financing the Education Role

Incremental Change

In principle, there is no reason that current GME funding under Medicare could not be more targeted to perceived health care workforce needs, as several states have done (Matherlee, 2001). DGME payments could be

---

[2] Numerous proposals for reform have been advanced in the literature but are not reviewed here. See, for example, Medicare Payment Advisory Commission, *Report to the Congress: Rethinking Medicare's Payment Policies for Graduate Medical Education and Teaching Hospitals*, Washington, DC: MedPAC, 1999. Anderson, G.F., G. Greenberg, and B. Wynn. "Graduate Medical Education: The Policy Debate" *Annu Rev Public Health* 22:35-47 (2001). Aaron, Henry (ed.), *The Future of Academic Medical Centers*, Washington, DC: Brookings Institution Press, 2001. Reports of The Commonwealth Fund Task Force on Academic Health Centers (www.cmwf.org).

restructured to encourage teaching institutions to train more geriatricians and other medical specialties in relatively short supply, and more nurses and other allied health professions. DGME could also be added onto other prospective payments, such as outpatient care or skilled nursing facility payments. Similarly, IME payments could be restructured to encourage teaching hospitals to train needed specialties and professions in the settings where they are most appropriately deployed. The add-on to inpatient DRG payments based on residents per bed could be replaced with other measures used as the basis for payment, that more directly track to society's health workforce needs. For example, training support for gerontologists could be linked to visits by older patients.

The advantage of this approach would be to make educational subsidy payments more consistent with technology and population trends, providing incentives to bring training into the community where more health care services are being delivered. Keeping the Medicare add-on structure in place would maintain the linkage with "automatic" entitlement funding.

The major disadvantage of this approach is it perpetuates the incongruity of trying to accomplish national health workforce objectives through Medicare reimbursement. It would also be more complex, requiring Congress and the Executive Branch to work together to establish objectives and implement them through changes to Medicare payment formulas, not a straightforward process. Finally, by maintaining the link with an entitlement program, this approach would be vulnerable to future budget cuts designed to control the growth of Medicare spending.

Fundamental Change

One major structural change would be to remove health workforce subsidization from Medicare and replace it with a separate program designed to formulate public goals and fund them directly. The program could be a separate entitlement that is linked to the achievement of national objectives or a separately authorized and appropriated "line item" in the federal budget, similar to the National Institutes of Health.

The advantage of a separate program would be to have national health workforce objectives supported by a national financing system. Once a national plan is formulated, institutions could be rewarded in proportion to their contribution to the achievement of national objectives. Additionally, the policy could be broadened to include all health professions receiving training in diverse settings, and adjusted periodically as perceptions of workforce needs change.

A disadvantage of this approach is that it would require some level of workforce planning, which may not fit American tastes. In addition, clinical education would have to compete with other budget priorities in the appropriations process, with uncertain outcome regarding the level of funding. This could be mediated with multiyear funding streams to provide some level of stability for the programs, yet permit periodic adjustments (similar to the funding of large, multiyear research studies). The uncertainty of year-to-year funding levels would be less of a problem if a new entitlement program were created. In this case, however, the beneficiaries of the program, and what they are entitled to, would need to be established. Whether appropriation or entitlement, creating such a fund would only address half the question; how the money is distributed, to whom, and for what purposes would also need to be addressed.

Financing the Research Role

Incremental Change

One approach to shrinking surplus patient care revenues and potentially reduced growth in government research sponsorship is to "broaden the base" of research undertakings to include more clinical research and to seek more opportunities for commercial support. NIH sponsorship may remain the mainstay of investigator-initiated research in AHCs, but it may also be supplemented with more clinical research, including that sponsored by private companies, to help cover the fixed costs of the research enterprise and secure new sources of revenue. AHCs might also place greater emphasis on making their technology transfer activities into profit-making enterprises by developing more of their discoveries into health care products, retaining property rights, and eventually adding to revenues through licensing and royalty fees.

The advantage of adopting this approach, which may already be under way in some institutions, is to reduce reliance on government-sponsored, basic science research funding sources and bring the research enterprise closer to the settings where health care is delivered. Doing so may help existing technologies to be utilized more effectively and earn a reputation for advancing technologies with the greatest potential for clinical application. These might include, of course, applications in genetics and proteomics and other leading-edge advances in modern medicine.

Disadvantages of this approach include potential dilution of the serendipitous discovery characterized by investigator-initiated research, and it would require more complex partnerships between scientific disciplines, including the social sciences, not often found in great numbers in AHCs. In addition, exploiting more private sector opportunities implies less freedom to independently pursue faculty research interests in AHCs.

Fundamental Change

Fundamental change in research could come from a shift in how priorities are set and by whom. As the availability of both old and new technologies grows and health care costs continue to rise, there will be increasing pressure on research institutions to provide more information on "what works, what doesn't, and at what cost" to aid in technology adoption and spending decisions. Payers, consumers, and regulators will have stronger input into the research agenda, in addition to the scientific community, with the potential to create a "sea change" in research priority setting within both public and private sectors. The Food and Drug Administration (FDA) and Center for Medicare & Medicaid Services (CMS) can expect to be pressured to include cost-effectiveness considerations in product approval and coverage decisions, respectively, and research enterprises (including NIH) will be pressured to place clinical research, including research on costs and benefits of new technology, on par with basic research. Improved coordination among funders, especially the federal funding agencies, could significantly affect priority setting for health-related research. Congressional action may be required to amend necessary statutes.

A change in research orientation of this magnitude would require AHCs and other research institutions to alter the mix of skills of personnel competing for, and performing, research to include more clinicians of various types and more social scientists. The resulting change in research focus would enable providers and payers to make more informed decisions regarding the deployment of medical technology and, possibly, to slow the pace at which new technology contributes to health care spending inflation. A disadvantage for AHCs would be a reorganization of how research gets done. AHCs would have to aggregate the skills and expertise to conduct clinical, health services, and prevention research. If they are unable to do this efficiently, the result could be a high proportion of such research being performed outside AHCs. More generally, a change in research priorities of this magnitude may slow the pace of discovery of new biomedical inventions and lose or delay their corresponding health benefits.

Financing the Patient Care Role

Incremental Change

As surplus revenues from insured services diminish, one incremental change that would provide greater support to safety net institutions would be to retarget Medicare and Medicaid DSH payments to institutions for uncompensated care to the uninsured and underinsured poor. Such payments could also be made to be less inpatient-focused by adding to reimbursement in different settings through formulas that directly measure uncompensated care rather than relying on proxy measures.

The advantage of this approach is that it would better target care subsidies to the greatest need. By doing so, it would remove the bias inherent in using Medicaid services as a proxy and help preserve institutions most relied upon for care to the poor. Disadvantages include continued reliance on entitlement programs to accomplish public policy concerning nonentitlement objectives, continued vulnerability to Medicare and Medicaid budget cuts, and potential difficulty in devising direct measures of uncompensated care that are unambiguously calculated and not subject to gaming.

Fundamental Change

If insurance programs, including Medicare, will become increasingly unwilling to subsidize the AHCs' roles, including uncompensated care, one rather dramatic solution is to enable all population segments to pay their own way, at least for some socially determined minimum standard of care. From a public policy standpoint, this means eliminating the uninsured either by providing them with insurance (or mandating insurance and providing subsidies based on financial and medical need) or by directly compensating providers for care to the uninsured (in essence, government is the insurer).

Advantages of this approach are to reduce unmet need and protect the institutions under pressure to find ways to fund uncompensated care. Attempts to widely broaden health insurance coverage have been tried, unsuccessfully, going back decades into the post-World War II, pre-Medicare era and, most recently, in the first Clinton term. One grave risk is that before we are able to get to a national solution to the uninsured, cost pressures may force some institutions to close and present serious access problems to the uninsured. So, a disadvantage of the nationalized approach to the uninsured is that it may require a dismantling of the safety net before we are able to get there politically. Also, its costs may be prohibitive.

IMPLICATIONS FOR THE FUTURE

AHCs can expect to face continued financial pressures in the future. Medicare will face continued stresses as the post-World War II "baby-boom" generation ages into the program and increases the volume of services that will be paid by it. At the same time, pressure is growing on Medicare to revise its benefits and include coverage for prescription medications. As demands for care increase and greater benefits are desired, the aging of the population is resulting in fewer workers paying into Social Security (relative to the size of the population over age 65) and, therefore, reduced funding for Medicare. The combination of these forces sounds an alarm for AHCs that rely on Medicare as a major source of funding for their activities, particularly for medical education that is funded through an entitlement.

Much of what is written in this chapter suggests that financing changes, through either natural evolution or public policy measures, will make it increasingly difficult for AHCs to cross-subsidize their roles by taking surplus revenues from insured patient services and applying them to shortfalls in education, research, and uncompensated care. It has been pointed out that because many of the costs of performing disparate roles are joint costs, it is impossible to determine what it costs to perform any single role with precision (Lewin, 2002; Vladeck, 2002). Nevertheless, it appears that financing trends are headed in the direction of making the roles performed by AHCs become "tubs on their own bottom."

The advantage of this trend, especially in gauging public subsidies, is transparency. If we "see" what it costs to pay for clinical education, for example, we are better able to gauge the necessity for, and returns to, public subsidy, and also to set goals and require accountability. On the other hand, if education and research, in particular, have to compete on a level playing field for public dollars at full cost, there may be fewer dollars available to pay for these roles than there would be under a system that relies heavily on cross-subsidization. The end result for some AHCs may be tough decisions that result in resizing their education and research enterprises.

Making all or some of these decisions will require that AHCs have better information on the resources and results of each of their roles toward improving health. Mission-based management is one approach for understanding the contribution of the various activities, but many schools have not budgeted systematically for their different activities performed (The Commonwealth Fund Task Force on Academic Health Centers, 2002). The Fund Flow Project of the University Healthcare Consortium is another approach to understanding the financial interdependencies between the component organizations of the AHC. AHCs will need to have systems in place to improve their understanding of the costs of each role, as well as the magnitude and direction of cross-subsidies in order to make the hard decisions with which they will be faced.

Financing policies will also need to change to support the innovative and collaborative approaches that AHCs are being asked to undertake in their roles. Research funders can do this by funding the collaborative, interdisciplinary approaches that can facilitate the development of knowledge across a whole continuum of research that includes not only discovery but also translation into care and evaluation. Payers for health services should be willing to support experimentation in both the delivery and the financing of care in order to develop processes of care that are safe, effective, and efficient, and that are designed to improve the health of patients and populations. Special attention should be given to improving care for underserved populations or to conditions that exhibit disparities in outcomes.

The committee believes that among all the AHC roles, the greatest pressure for change will be in the education role. Chapter 3 described the need for significant reform in the content and methods of clinical education, and this chapter described the current and projected pressures on its financing. Whereas funding for research has been expanding, support for education has been contracting. The education reforms that AHCs are being asked to undertake are of sufficient magnitude that organizations will undoubtedly face costs in retooling their programs.

Funding for education needs to support needed reforms and should be made available immediately for this purpose. Either new funds should be provided or existing resources be redirected. If existing resources are redirected, the options are to redirect a portion of DGME or a portion of IME. As noted before, DGME covers Medicare's share of the hospital's expenses for resident stipends, faculty salaries, and related expenses. IME payments are provided as an add-on to the hospital's DRG payments to support the additional costs of caring for Medicare patients that are attributable to teaching activities. For example, extra tests may be performed as students learn, staffing levels may be higher because of the demands placed on other hospital staff, or patients at teaching hospitals may be sicker than is accounted for in the case mix index. These increase the costs of treating Medicare patients in teaching hospitals.

Analyses by the Medicare Payment Advisory Commission (MedPAC) found that Medicare's IME adjustment formula is about twice the calculated estimate of the relationship between teaching intensity and the increased costs of patient care (MedPAC, 2002). It is has been recognized for some time that the actual adjustment for IME is higher than the statistical estimates. Congress made an explicit decision to approximately double the IME factor at the time that the prospective payment system (PPS) was being put in place for hospitals because they were concerned about its impact on academic health centers. When Congress originally passed the PPS provisions in 1983, the amount provided for IME was 11.6 percent for each 10 percent increase in a hospital's ratio of residents to beds. Since then, the rate has been reduced multiple times to reach a level of 5.5 percent for 2003 and beyond (MedPAC, 2001; Matherlee, 2001). Analyses have found that the effect of medical education on patient care costs has decreased, due to combined improvements in the Medicare case-mix index, the DRG patient classification system, and the relative efficiency of major teaching hospitals (Lave, 2001).

For 2003, MedPAC estimates that about 2.5 percentage points of the 5.5 percent IME add-on, or about $2.5 billion, are in excess of the current cost relationship (MedPAC, 2002). The Council on Graduate Medical Education has recommended that IME payments be set at no more than the analytically justified level for teaching activities (COGME, 2000). At its January 2003 meeting, MedPAC identified the need to continue to study possibilities for better targeting of IME funds (MedPAC, 2003).

Rather than reducing the level of IME, the amount that exceeds the relationship between teaching and Medicare patient care costs could be redirected to explicitly support reforms in education. This would bring the IME factor in line with estimate of the increased costs of patient care associated with teaching activities, as it is intended to do, and provide a means to jump start the process of education reform. As noted in chapter 3, educational reform will entail much more than just changing curricula, but will also include changes in the care settings in which education takes place, so the use of IME funds for educational reform is also consistent with its intent.

Although immediate reforms in individual educational programs can be supported, the committee believes that long-term, more broadly based changes in the financing of education will also be required. This chapter has already described the problems and gaps in current financing methods for clinical education and its ability to respond to future needs of the population. Proposals have been put forward to create a fund, with contributions from all payers, to support medical education (COGME, 2000; The Commonwealth Task Force on Academic Health Centers, 1997a). Although such proposals have offered guidance on alternatives for creating a pool of funds, less consideration has been given to how such funds should be disbursed. For example, should there be a relationship to broader workforce goals, are there desired attributes that training programs must demonstrate (e.g., use of nonhospital or interdisciplinary approaches), is there a relationship between the training of physician and nonphysician clinicians, who should be the recipient of funds, or what might be mechanisms of accountability.

Alternative approaches might also be explored. For example, the cancer centers program of the National Cancer Institute requires different responsibilities from three levels of cancer centers and provides different amounts of core support (although the percentage of support is equal).[3]

---

[3]Three types of centers are recognized, with varying scope of activities. *Comprehensive cancer centers* conduct basic, clinical, and prevention/behavioral/population-based research, and perform outreach and education to the health professionals and people in the community

The corollary in clinical education would be the presence of three types of education programs, such as those in AHCs, major teaching hospitals, and other teaching hospitals, each with varying scopes of education programs. Additional work would be needed to explore whether and how such a model would have applicability to clinical education, but it illustrates the possibility of alternative approaches.

If AHCs are being asked to innovate across all of their roles to meet the changing needs and demands of the future, financing policies will also need to support, encourage, and facilitate such innovation.

---

served. *Clinical cancer centers* conduct at least clinical research and may do other research as well. *Cancer centers* conduct research in a narrowly defined area, such as population research. Core funding, set at 20 percent of the NCI-supported research program at the institution, supports infrastructure and developmental work. Centers obtain program funds through the competitive NIH grant process. Centers are evaluated every five years. (The Cancer Centers Branch of the National Cancer Institute, www3.cancer.gov and personal communication, Brian Kimes and Linda Weiss, September 27, 2002).

CHAPTER 7

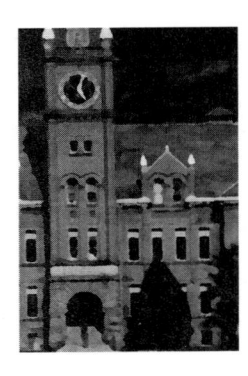

Expectations for the AHC of the 21st Century

Previous chapters of this report have reviewed how the external environment in which AHCs function will change in very fundamental ways in the future, affecting how AHCs carry out each of their roles both individually and in combination. Nonetheless, the AHC roles in education, research, and patient care will remain important in the future. The public will continue to need a well-prepared workforce, to value the discoveries science can offer, and to seek innovations in the delivery of care. However, it is also true that each role will require modification and adaptation to meet the needs of the 21st century. Because the roles remain relevant does not imply that their execution and approach need not change.

This chapter synthesizes the discussion and findings of preceding chapters to provide a set of recommendations for each role performed by AHCs, with emphasis on how each will need to be transformed to meet the needs of the public in the coming decades. The AHC of the 21st century will need to use its roles, resources, and leadership to improve the health of patients and populations. To this end, it will have to lead in the development, refinement, and application of the evidence base and education grounded in the evidence base as the foundation for both treating illness and improving health. In the committee's vision of the 21st century AHC, AHCs will effectively integrate their roles so that research develops the evidence base, patient care applies and refines the evidence base, and education teaches evidence-based care, and all are designed in an overall context of and commitment to improving health.

TRANSFORMING THE ROLES OF THE 21ST-CENTURY AHC

The prior chapters in this report have identified a number of forces for change in the environment within which AHCs carry out their roles. Because AHCs are major participants in each of these roles, the challenge of transforming the roles to respond to this changing environment falls particularly to them, although all organizations performing any of the roles should also meet the expectations for each. The modifications required have been described in previous chapters and are summarized in Table 7-1.

AHCs need to respond to the forces for change, and the nation has the right to look to them for such a response. AHCs need to respond for several reasons. The forces for change described in Chapter 2 are more likely to increase, not lessen in the coming years. The population will continue to age and diversify, and the pace of technological change will increase. The rising costs of care threaten AHCs in a number of ways. State budget crises have caused some states to question their support for graduate medical education and to consider its withdrawal or reduction. Rising costs can be expected in turn to increase the number of uninsured, many of whom rely on AHCs for their care. To the extent that higher costs of care affect hospital operating margins, access to capital will also be affected. The pressures on AHCs can be expected to intensify, rather than lessen, in the future.

Although AHCs have successfully represented their concerns at the federal and state levels in the past, it will probably be more difficult to count on continued relief in the coming years. Emerging concerns are reordering priorities as concerns with deficits, bioterrorism and homeland security, Medicare reform, and malpractice are reordering priorities as they draw the attention of policy makers. Furthermore, if AHCs are unable to demonstrate sufficient progress in meeting society's changing and emerging needs (as described in previous chapters), future support is likely to come with increasing legislative or regulatory restrictions, which could potentially leave AHCs with fewer options to respond. The sooner AHCs act, the better chance they will have of controlling their future.

The nation has a right to expect AHCs to respond because the way in which AHCs carry out their activities in education, research, and patient care influences the capabilities that reside throughout the health system generally. Although all health care organizations are affected by the trends described in this report, the choices made by AHCs will have an effect well beyond their own organizations, exerting a profound influence on what kind of health care the American people will enjoy. Decisions about how to train health professionals influence the clinical skills they use in practicing within the larger system. Decisions about what types of research to pursue and how to share the results influence future practice patterns and insurance policies.

TABLE 7-1 Adapting the Roles of AHCs

Role	20th Century	21st Century
Education	Education that emphasized: • Treatment of symptoms of individual patients • Activities of individual practitioners • Hospital-based training • Undergraduate and graduate training	Education that emphasizes: • Teaching of research-based best practices in a variety of clinical settings that model best practices • Understanding of the determinants of health and illness • Use of evidence-based educational methods • Coordination of approaches across the continuum of education and across clinical and management education
Patient Care	Patient care that emphasized: • Treatment of the symptoms and illnesses of patients who arrive at the institution • Relative emphasis on specialty care • Care that reflects predominantly local patterns of practice	Patient care that emphasizes: • Development of structures and team approaches designed to improve health • Modeling, testing, and refinement of research-based best practices for clinical care • Use of collaborative approaches to health, especially for vulnerable populations
Research	Research that emphasized: • Basic research advances • Accomplishments of an individual principal investigator • Publication in professional journals	Research that emphasizes: • Linking of basic, clinical, health services, and prevention research • Improved understanding of the clinical, organizational, and cost effectiveness of new treatments and established practices • Teams of researchers that span the sciences • Translation of knowledge into practice

Additionally, AHCs receive a significant level of public support for their activities. Over the last decade, the federal and state governments have allocated approximately $100 billion to support activities in clinical education and research and to provide disproportionate-share funds to care for the poor and uninsured (Anderson, 2002).[1] The majority of this funding

---

[1] These are estimates for the AHC enterprise. It is recognized that Medicare funds for graduate medical education are provided to the hospital, whereas much of the National Institutes of Health (NIH) funding goes to individual investigators at the medical, nursing, or other professional school.

has gone to support the activities of AHCs, so the nation has the right to look to them for guidance and leadership in addressing the health needs of the American people.

Finally, the current health care system is characterized by many problems, such as the increasing costs of care, dissatisfaction on the part of both patients and those working in health care, and evidence of disparities in health, as well as clear opportunities to improve health status. Recent surveys revealed that 79 percent of the public and 83 percent of physicians believed the health care system needed fundamental change or a complete rebuilding (Blendon et al., 2001). Another study found that 41 percent of hospital nurses were dissatisfied with their jobs, and 23 percent planned to leave their jobs within the next year (Aiken et al., 2001). Because of the complexity of the problems facing the system, no single solution will suffice; in any case, however, AHCs need to be a part of the solution for improving the health care system.

The prior six chapters have documented the need for change in how AHCs carry out their roles if they are to continue to serve the public interest in the coming decades. The aim of the committee's proposed overall strategy for accomplishing this transformation is to start a process of continuing and long-term change. The recommendations that follow offer a two-part plan. First, the external environment should create a set of incentives that will clearly signal the need for change in each of the AHC roles and serve as a spur for actions by the AHCs. In education, Congress should create a dedicated fund that can foster innovation in the educational approaches used to prepare health professionals. In research, federal funding agencies should work together to support collaborations among a mix of scientists that do different types of research, to answer the big questions of science and health. In patient care, public and private payers and foundations should support experimentation in working across settings of care to redesign and restructure care processes that are aimed at improving the health of both patients and populations.

In response to the external changes described in this report, AHCs should examine how they carry out their roles and adapt them as necessary. In education, AHCs will need to examine fundamentally the methods and approaches used to prepare health professionals; adapting current curricula will not be sufficient. In research, AHCs will need to examine how their research programs link across the continuum of research; expanding the number of studies done will not be sufficient. In patient care, AHCs will need to restructure care processes to focus on health for patients and populations; improving institutionally based care for their own patients will not be sufficient.

The second part of the proposed strategy addresses the AHC itself, rather than any specific role, and asks AHCs to examine how they organize, perform, assess, and internally support their varied roles. The recommendations offered to this end call on AHCs to establish systems across the enterprise that will facilitate the flow of information throughout the AHC, foster accountability to measure and reward needed changes, and develop leaders who will take on the transformations required.

It is not possible to assign any given recommendation to the medical or nursing school, to the AHC hospital, or to any other individual component of the overall AHC. Given the interdependence of the AHC roles, no individual component of the AHC can accomplish any given recommendation. For example, the medical school can reform its own curriculum but cannot unilaterally achieve more interdisciplinary approaches in education unless it works with the nursing, public health, allied health, and other schools. Educators can reform a curriculum but must work closely with clinical faculty in the hospital or other practice sites to affect the training experience for students. Improving and accelerating the translation of research into clinical care will require close work between the professional schools and the hospitals and clinics. Furthermore, because AHCs are organized in different ways, the committee believes it is not possible to assign selected recommendations to specific components of the AHC in a way that would be meaningful for all AHCs.

Implementing the committee's recommendations will require that AHCs function as a more coordinated and cohesive operating entity across their constellation of organizations and functions. AHCs have traditionally described themselves as having multiple roles—in research, in education, and in patient care. As long as AHCs view these roles as separate and distinct, the aim will be to maximize each, a perspective that creates a set of conflicts. There is a trade-off, for example, between the AHCs' research and patient care roles. As research organizations, the AHCs are objective arbiters of what does and does not work in health care (Thier, 1994), but as competitors in the clinical services market, they want to use a new procedure or technology before others do so, sometimes in advance of full knowledge on its effectiveness. There is also a trade-off between the education and patient care roles. As educators, AHCs have as a primary goal providing health professionals with a broad-based education that recognizes the whole patient and the factors that affect health and illness; patient care in the acute care setting is episodic, with a procedural and specialty focus. The more specialized an AHC's services become, the less representative are its patients, and this in turn compromises its effectiveness as a training site. Finally, there is a similar trade-off between the education and research roles in that research questions tend to be defined to test hypotheses, whereas the education of health professionals should provide a broad understanding of the processes of health and illness. In economic terms, each activity has a different production function (Samuelson and Nordhaus, 1989).

Furthermore, maximizing each role will not necessarily lead to improvements in health. Maximizing the number of specialists trained may not produce better health, maximizing the number of research studies conducted may not translate into better care for people; and maximizing the number of physician visits or hospital admissions may not affect health status.

AHCs should recognize the interdependent and complementary nature of their historically individual roles within an overall context that encompasses a commitment to improving the health of patients and populations. Indeed, the unique contribution of AHCs in coming decades will lie in their ability to achieve such an integration of their roles within medicine and across all health sciences, including public health, nursing, dentistry, pharmacy, and others, to foster the health of all Americans. By effectively capitalizing on opportunities for integration across roles, specialties, and professions, AHCs could potentially improve health outcomes, accelerate the translation of scientific discoveries into safe and effective practices, lead the way toward more efficient use of human capital and technology, improve public health, and promote healthy lifestyles. This integration involves more than the simultaneous provision of education, research, and patient care. It requires the purposeful linkage of these roles so that research develops the evidence base, patient care applies and refines the evidence base, and education teaches evidence-based approaches to care and prevention.

The title of this report calls on AHCs to lead efforts for change. Leading such efforts for the 21st century will require that AHCs initiate change within and across their roles, as well as throughout their own diverse organizations.

RECOMMENDATIONS

Before providing its recommendations, the committee wishes to emphasize its serious concern regarding the problems facing people who are uninsured, recognizing the relationship among a lack of insurance, difficulties in accessing care, and an individual's health (Institute of Medicine, 2001a, 2002). AHCs that care for a disproportionate share of the poor and uninsured bear a financial burden that may affect their ability to continue to carry out their core activities in research and education. The committee has not made a specific recommendation regarding this problem because its impact is broader than AHCs. Furthermore, the committee recognizes that the consequences for AHCs of a program that offers universal coverage, such as national health insurance, are unclear, and depend on how cost containment efforts or support for research and education might be structured. However, we strongly urge that the ranks of the uninsured be reduced, and that AHCs devote more of their attention to the future challenges of improving the health and well-being of all people.

The committee believes that among all the AHC roles, education will require the greatest changes in the coming decades, and our recommendations in this area are quite specific. We regard education as one of the primary mechanisms for initiating a cultural shift toward an emphasis on the needs of patients and populations and a focus on improving health, using the best of science and the best of caring. Thus, our recommendations start with this role.

Transforming the Roles of AHCs for the 21st Century

Reforming the Education of Health Professionals

AHCs have historically emphasized the education of physicians at the undergraduate and graduate levels, relying on the hospital's inpatient and outpatient settings as primary training sites. Guiding the education role so that it prepares health professionals not just to treat illnesses of patients but to have an impact on the health of populations will require much more than curricular change. Rather, a more fundamental review of the approaches, methods, and settings used in clinical education will be required.

Recommendation 1: AHCs should take the lead in reforming the content and methods of health professions education to include the integrated development of educational curricula and approaches that:

a. Enable and encourage coordination among deans of various professional schools and leaders across disciplines (such as medicine, dentistry, nursing, public health, pharmacy, social work, and basic sciences) to remove internal barriers to interprofessional education.

b. Ensure that all teaching environments—from the classroom to sites for clinical rotations and preceptorships and practice—are exemplars for the future of health care delivery (e.g., by modeling team-based care and using information technology) and, in collaboration with local health care leaders, demonstrate how to improve health for populations and communities, as well as individual patients.

c. Emphasize training in skills that will be needed to improve health, such as the theory and computational skills necessary to comprehend the new biological sciences, as well as the social and behavioral sciences.

d. Develop, recognize, and reward those who teach and conduct research on clinical education.

Health professions training is a major factor in creating the culture and attitudes that will guide a lifetime of practice; however, health care practitioners will not be prepared for practice in the 21st century without fundamental changes in the approaches, methods, and settings used for all levels of clinical education. Current training of health professionals emphasizes primarily the biological basis of disease and treatment of symptoms, with insufficient attention to the social, behavioral, and other factors that contribute to healing and are part of creating healthy populations. The training of disciplines in separate "silos" creates boundaries where coordination and collaboration are needed to improve health. Furthermore, there is little coordination among undergraduate, graduate, and continuing education; the result is duplication in some areas and gaps in others.

If care is to be more patient-centered, focus on improving the health of people, and meet the needs of an aging, chronically ill, and increasingly diverse population, educational programs will require major redesign and reorientation to integrate training across the disciplines, adequately prepare and reward educators, and conduct research to expand the evidence base on health professions education. Furthermore, the clinical setting in which students are taught must be able to demonstrate care that is patient-centered and health-improving, and model practices that are evidence-based, continuously improving, and cost-efficient. For example, it is meaningless to teach the importance of interdisciplinary teams or the use of clinical information systems if such approaches are not exemplified in the practice settings in which students are taught.

Although curricular changes will be required, adding one more course to an already overcrowded curriculum is not the answer. New approaches to clinical education will be required, especially to reflect practice in interdisciplinary teams and greater use of information and communications systems. Although educational reform is being undertaken in most disciplines, more such efforts are needed, not only within but also across disciplines, since changes by one group of practitioners will affect the work of others.

AHCs should take a leadership role in reforming clinical education. In addition, education oversight organizations (accrediting, licensing, and certifying bodies) should work together and revise their standards to require demonstration of competencies in patient-centered care, interdisciplinary teams, evidence-based practice, quality improvement, and informatics, as called for in a recent Institute of Medicine report (Institute of Medicine, 2003). Finally, funders must send a clear signal that these types of changes in health professions education are important and must happen more quickly, as urged in the next recommendation.

Recommendation 2: Congress should support innovation in clinical education through changes in the financing of clinical education.

a. Congress should create an ongoing fund that provides competitive grants to support educational innovation.

- Funds should support educational innovations such as use of clinical information systems, testing of new educational approaches in hospital and nonhospital settings, and evaluation of curricular and other needed reforms in clinical education. Priority for such funds should be given to those organizations that integrate the training of multiple health disciplines (e.g., medicine, nursing, pharmacy, therapy, public health, administration) and that use information technology in their clinical education programs.

- To create this education innovation fund, Congress should redirect the portion of the funding provided for indirect medical education that exceeds the additional costs of caring for Medicare patients that are attributable to teaching activities (commonly referred to as the "empirical amount"). Availability of these funds should be contingent upon implementing innovations in clinical education and training environments.

b. In addition, Congress and the administration should promptly revise the current statutory framework of Medicare support for graduate medical education to support more interdisciplinary, team-based, nonhospital training that aims to improve the health of patients and populations. Revisions should include consideration of whether other payers should provide specific support for the education of health professionals; examine the relationship between support for the training of physician and nonphysician clinicians; assess the appropriate recipient of support; and identify mechanisms for accountability for both the disbursement and the use of public funds.

The committee recommends a two-pronged approach to address both short- and long-term issues in the financing of clinical education. First, the recommended innovation fund should be created using a portion of the public resources currently devoted to existing programs to initiate immediate change in individual training programs. AHCs need to make changes in the content, methods, and approaches for clinical education, and support should be provided for those efforts through the innovation fund.

Second, a set of more broad-based, long-lasting changes is also needed. The committee does not question continued support for health professions education but believes that the current methods are insufficient to meet future needs and must be fundamentally revised to encourage the training of a workforce that will be prepared to work in the interdisciplinary, health-oriented, information-driven models of care of the 21st century. Current funding methods for clinical education do not adequately support training in nonhospital settings, foster interdisciplinary approaches to training, or consider the relationship between the training of physician and nonphysician clinicians. The methods have encouraged growth in the number, size, and duration of medical residency programs and the training of specialists in inpatient tertiary settings (Henderson, 2000; Young and Coffman, 1998). For nurses and allied health professionals (including, for example, physician assistants), current payment methods have favored programs in settings that do not train physicians and are not linked to universities. Current policies do not give either AHCs or Medicare the flexibility or encouragement to make adjustments as workforce needs change, even when clear needs are identified, such as clinicians to care for an aging, chronically ill population. State and federal policy makers continue to struggle with persistent problems regarding the mix and distribution of health professionals. The changes needed are large enough to require a fuller examination of the approaches used and incentives created by current funding mechanisms.

As noted in Chapter 6, a number of prior proposals for revising payment for clinical education have been advanced. The committee believes a broad view is needed, one that considers the development of the workforce required for the future. This analysis should move forward promptly while the innovation fund supports immediate changes that AHCs can and clearly should be developing.

The committee identified three options for creating an education innovation fund. One was to create a new funding program. The education of health professionals is of sufficient value to society to justify the allocation of new funds to such an endeavor. Another option was to freeze current payments for graduate medical education and channel the amount due to inflation that would occur under the existing program into the innovation fund. Using this mechanism, about $40 million would have been made available to such a fund in 2001.[2]

The third option was to redirect a portion of the current funding for indirect medical education (IME) to reforms in clinical education. IME payments to teaching hospitals are intended to support the additional costs of caring for Medicare patients that are attributable to teaching activities. Analyses by the Medicare Payment Advisory Commission (MedPAC) revealed that Medicare's IME adjustment formula for 2002 is about twice the

---

[2]This figure assumes that $2 billion was provided to hospitals for direct medical education costs and that the Consumer Price Index was 2 percent.

calculated estimate of these higher costs (Medicare Payment Advisory Commission, 2002). For 2003, MedPAC estimates that about 2.5 percentage points of the 5.5 percent IME add-on (about $2.6 billion) is in excess of the current cost relationship (Medicare Payment Advisory Commission, 2003). These funds go into a hospital's general revenues, with no requirements placed on their use. AHCs use these funds to support other mission-related activities, so their use varies across AHCs. In its March 2003 report to Congress, MedPAC expressed its dissatisfaction with current payment policy because there is no accountability for the use of funds beyond the amount associated with the higher patient care costs attributable to teaching activities (Medicare Payment Advisory Commission, 2003).

The committee does not deem it likely that an entirely new funding source could be created and does not believe that redirecting the increment provided by inflation would provide sufficient funds to support the endeavor. Using a portion of the IME add-on would produce a larger pool of funds to support educational innovation.

The committee believes that as the primary funder of graduate medical education, Medicare has a responsibility to send a clear signal on the need for change in these programs. Medicare should exercise this responsiblity because the program needs to ensure the availability of an adequately prepared workforce that is able to meet the health needs of the Medicare population, such as the provision of effective and efficient care to maintain and improve the health of people with chronic conditions. Furthermore, as noted previously, making these types of changes in clinical education will affect patient care. It can be assumed, therefore, that the changes will also affect the costs of treating Medicare patients in teaching hospitals, which is the intended purpose of providing the IME percentage add-on.

Redirecting a portion of the funds currently provided for IME is intended to spur or accelerate the process of change in clinical education. By structuring this as a grant program, AHCs would have to describe how the funds would be used to make the types of changes called for in this report. The aim is to motivate the necessary discussions across the schools, disciplines, faculty, and organizations within the AHC. As noted previously, making changes in one role will require adaptations in other roles (e.g., modeling best practices in training programs will require evaluating the application of evidence-based practice in current patient care processes). Therefore, the proposed innovation fund could provide an incentive for AHCs to examine the design of and approaches to clinical education, and also foster the types of discussion and decision making throughout the AHC enterprise that will be necessary to undertake changes in the AHCs' education and other roles.

AHCs are concerned about diminishing support for IME, so it is important to recognize that the committee does not recommend a reduction of overall support to AHCs. Rather, our recommendation directs that AHCs have the opportunity to retain the funds and that Medicare have the opportunity to send a strong signal for change while inserting a level of accountability for the use of those funds. Administering the innovation fund through a grant program involves a mechanism at which AHCs are both adept and successful. Although the committee's recommendation does not represent a loss of funds to AHCs, it could result in a loss of flexibility in the use of the funds in that they would be disbursed through a grant program rather than payment for services. To the extent that an AHC uses IME funds to subsidize care to the uninsured, for example, there is a risk that such services could be curtailed. However, there is a weak relationship between those teaching hospitals that receive IME funds and those that provide the most care to the poor and uninsured (Medicare Payment Advisory Commission, 2003; Anderson et al., 2001). It would be appropriate for the Centers for Medicare and Medicaid Services and MedPAC to monitor carefully the effects of the establishment of the innovation fund for any deleterious effects.

Demonstrating New Models of Care

Changing health needs and changing technologies create both demands and opportunities for new models of care that are designed to treat illnesses of patients as well as improve the health of populations. As centers of education for health professionals, AHCs must ensure that the care they deliver is designed to improve health and model the best evidence-based, continuously improving, cost-efficient practices for students, practitioners in the community, and the community at large.

Recommendation 3: AHCs should design and assess new structures and approaches for patient care.

a. AHCs should work across disciplines and, where appropriate, across settings of care in their communities to develop organizational structures and team approaches designed to improve health. Such approaches should be incorporated into clinical education to teach health-oriented processes of care.

b. Public and private payers, state and federal agencies, and foundations should provide support for demonstration projects designed to test and evaluate the organizational structures and team approaches designed to improve health and prevent disease. Demonstrations should target in particular (1) populations that are at high risk for serious illness, (2) populations that are financially vulnerable, (3) conditions that reflect disparities across the population, and (4) methods for supporting individuals' involvement in and decisions about their health. Demonstrations should encompass both financing and delivery components, including the testing of organizational reforms that optimize work design and workforce management. Payers should streamline the process for incorporating successful demonstration results into coverage and payment policies.

As the health needs of people change and the health care system's capabilities expand, the potential to improve health will grow. Improved processes of care have been shown to improve health and reduce costs for chronically ill populations, for the frail elderly, and for uninsured populations (Wagner et al., 1996; Bodenheimer et al., 2002; Wieland et al., 2000; Kaufman et al., 2000). But, for the most part, current processes of care are not designed to realize that potential (Institute of Medicine, 2001b).

Developing structures and approaches that can improve the health not only of patients but also of populations will require AHCs both to examine critically the processes of care within their own care settings and to reach out to their surrounding communities to collaborate with other providers and services (including complementary and alternative health services) and with public health agencies. Within their own setting, AHCs will need to examine how to improve systems of service and care to make them safer and more effective and efficient. Technological advances and the changing composition of the health care workforce will permit new work designs and require that models of care improve not only quality, but also productivity. AHCs should be using their patient care settings to test organizational reforms that can optimize work design and workforce management (including evidence-based management), thereby increasing retention of health professionals and reducing dissatisfaction with the work environment.

It is important that AHCs take on the role of demonstrating new models of care because their patient care setting is where research and education intersect. As the committee envisions the 21st century AHC, it will develop the evidence base that is applied in patient care and then demonstrate good patterns of practice to students.

Since improved processes of care will also benefit those who pay for care, public payers (such as the Centers for Medicare and Medicaid Services and state Medicaid programs) and private payers (such as insurance companies and managed care organizations) need to encourage and support innovations aimed at redesigning care to improve health. The committee recommends that demonstration projects to be funded include both financing and delivery innovations so payers can use the results and facilitate their replication in other practice settings.

Both public and private payers have undertaken such efforts in some areas. The Centers for Medicare and Medicaid Services has sponsored demonstration projects in a variety of areas, such as experimentation in developing new models of care in disease management, case management, and coordinated care, and AHCs have participated in these efforts (Berenson and Horvath, 2003; Centers for Medicare and Medicaid Services, 2003). Aetna is sponsoring a series of initiatives to assess and track racial and ethnic disparities in health care and is providing grants to identify and test means of reducing or eliminating disparities in health status and delivery of health care, providing funds for the purpose to AHCs such as the Johns Hopkins University and the University of Michigan (Aetna, 2003). Along these same lines, the National Institutes of Health (NIH) has also provided support to Columbia University to develop a center on minority health and health disparities. This center will establish community collaborations aimed at understanding how access to care shapes disparities in health care use and outcomes and develop a 4-year cultural competency curriculum for medical students (Association of American Medical Colleges, 2003).

The committee believes more such efforts are needed. One of the challenges involved is that payers may not realize the benefits from their investments if the benefits accrue to the population at large or appear only after many years. A recently released report by the Institute of Medicine calls for bold, large-scale demonstrations to test new approaches for health care financing and delivery that are able to link the delivery and public health systems and focus on improving population health while eliminating disparities (Institute of Medicine, 2002e). Another Institute of Medicine report notes the need for demonstration projects focused on improving care provided to the chronically ill by redesigning care delivery across multiple providers, supporting patient self-management, and implementing community-wide education efforts to improve population health (Institute of Medicine, 2003).

Translating the Discoveries of Science into Improved Health

AHCs have been significant contributors to the enormous strides made in research in recent years. The challenge in the coming decades will be to apply those advances and new laboratory discoveries to clinical settings and community practices so their benefits will reach more people.

Recommendation 4: Health-related research needs to span the continuum from discovery to testing to application and evaluation.

a. AHCs should increase their emphasis on clinical, health services, prevention, community-based, and translational research that can move basic discoveries into clinical and community settings.

b. Congress and the administration should coordinate funding across agencies that support health-related research including the life sciences (biomedical, clinical, health services, and prevention research), the physical sciences, and other sciences that advance health. More coordinated funding efforts and the criteria for evaluating funding support should foster interdisciplinary and collaborative arrangements that cut across departments, professional schools, and institutions.

To improve health, it will be necessary in the coming decades to place an increased emphasis on clinical, health services, and prevention research so the discoveries of basic science can be translated into improved health care for people. Clinical and health services research can help answer questions in a variety of areas, including the clinical, organizational, and cost effectiveness of new therapies as well as current practices; effective methods for promoting healthy behaviors; the design of safe, cost-efficient, and effective processes of care; and methods for incorporating best practices into various clinical settings. Increased attention should also be paid to prevention research, which can also have a translational aspect in enhancing our understanding of what works and what does not work in prevention and of the interaction between personal health and population health. In addition to translating basic scientific discoveries into clinical applications, greater priority should be given to how organizations can translate the findings of health services research into institutional and other settings.

Asking AHCs to conduct research across the continuum and establish priorities does not mean asking every AHC to expand its research activities. Historically, AHCs have focused on basic biomedical research, with support from the NIH, primarily provided to individual investigators. AHCs have emphasized in particular basic scientific research, a foundation for the health-related "research and development" activities that make future advances possible. The committee is asking the AHCs to consider research needs across the continuum, assess their resources and capabilities, review their current and projected research portfolios, and set priorities within an overall context of improving health. Furthermore, AHCs will need to examine how their research activities are organized throughout the enterprise. The approaches used in conducting clinical, health services, and prevention research tend to be interdisciplinary, and the conduct of such research can be difficult within an AHC structure and operating system built around departments. In addition, the involvement of human participants in research often raises bioethical concerns and/or conflicts of interest, issues that require attention at the level of both the individual investigator and the organization (Gelijns and Thier, 2002; Boyd and Bero, 2000; Institute of Medicine, 2001, 2002b).

It is important to maintain strong support for basic research to sustain continued scientific advances, but research funders will also need to consider how they can support the types of collaborations needed for translating discoveries into practice. In the future, significant scientific advances are likely to result from interdisciplinary approaches that involve a mix of sciences and scientists. Understanding the application of genetics, for example, will require basic research to understand the mechanisms, but also clinical and prevention research to apply the results to patients and populations, attention to issues of organizational design so providers can deliver the care, an understanding of costs and financing to build its use into the health system, and a focus on how to educate patients and professionals so everyone understands the potential and limitations of the science. Yet each of these matters is addressed by different scientists who are funded separately, and usually by different agencies. Research in the newer sciences will require crossing boundaries that were created in the past, bringing biologists, chemists, physicists, engineers, and mathematicians together with a mix of clinical and other investigators to work together in the laboratory and other research settings. Additionally, research aimed at improving health will require more extensive collaborations involving not only those in the fields of medicine and public health, but also behavioral and social scientists, communications specialists, and others.

Research funders can influence greatly whether and how linkages are made across the continuum of research so that knowledge is developed and able to reach those who can benefit. For example, the cancer centers program of the National Cancer Institute supports broad-based, interdisciplinary programs of research characterized by the ability to integrate a diversity of research approaches, aimed at influencing standards of care and ultimately reducing cancer incidence, morbidity, and mortality (National Cancer Institute, 2002).[3] Comprehensive cancer centers conduct a range of research, including basic, clinical, and preventative/ behavioral/population-based research, as well as outreach, education, and dissemination. Another

---

[3]Three types of centers are recognized, with varying scopes of activity. *Comprehensive cancer centers* conduct basic, clinical, and preventative/behavioral/population-based research, and provide outreach and education to health professionals and others in the community served. *Clinical cancer centers* conduct at least clinical research and may do other research as well. *Cancer centers* conduct research in a narrowly defined area, such as population research. Core funding, set at 20 percent of the National Cancer Institute–supported research program at the institution, supports infrastructure and developmental work. Centers obtain program funds through the competitive NIH grant process and are evaluated every 5 years (Cancer Centers Branch of the National Cancer Institute, www3.cancer.gov/cancercenters/, and personal communication with Brian Kimes and Linda Weiss, National Cancer Institute, September 27, 2002).

example is the Framingham Heart Study, sponsored by NIH since 1948 (in association since 1971 with an AHC, Boston University), which has produced much of what is known today about the risk of cardiovascular disease (National Heart, Lung and Blood Institute, 2003). Examples such as these can provide a framework for efforts across agencies.

Improved communication, coordination, and opportunities for interagency funding for both programmatic and training support should enable the types of collaboration needed to answer the questions of science and health likely to be most important in the coming decades. Although some interagency funding efforts are in place, coordination would be required at the federal level among NIH, the Centers for Disease Control and Prevention, the Health Resources and Services Administration, the Agency for Healthcare Research and Quality, the Centers for Medicare and Medicaid Services, the Food and Drug Administration, the Veterans Health Administration, the Department of Defense, the Department of Energy, the Environmental Protection Agency, the National Science Foundation, and even the National Aeronautics and Space Administration (National Science and Technology Council, 2000).

This chapter has presented a series of recommendations pertaining to each role performed by AHCs. Because of the interdependencies across these roles, it is difficult to change one role without affecting the others. Furthermore, rather than layering more activities over current ones and overloading a faculty that is already thinly stretched, implementing the recommendations in this chapter will require action and leadership at the level of the overall AHC. The next and final chapter of this report identifies three strategic management systems that all AHCs will have to address: (1) making greater use of information and communications technology to manage information and knowledge across the entire AHC enterprise, (2) establishing goals for change at the AHC-wide level and measuring performance against those goals, and (3) developing and supporting leaders within the AHC who are able to guide the changes described in this report and lead the nation in health.

CHAPTER 8

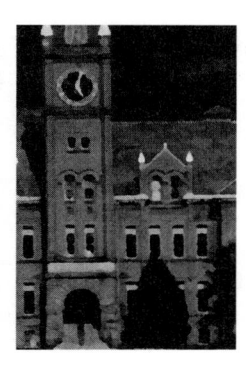

CREATING SYSTEMS FOR CHANGE IN AHCs

The prior chapter presented four recommendations for altering the direction of the AHC roles to meet the new demands of the coming decades. The complexity of the AHCs' organizational structures and their mix of roles pose a dilemma in how to approach these four recommendations.

Organizationally, an AHC is essentially a conglomeration of organizations. Most AHCs function like a holding company, a central entity that loosely supports and coordinates the component organizations (Zelman et al., 1999). The component organizations grew under separate governance and have generally pursued their own individual objectives, with a minimum of central management and oversight (Norlin and Osborn, 1998; Korn, 1996). The AHC roles are performed at different places in the institution and have to satisfy different customers. Clinical care is the primary focus of the hospital and faculty practice plans. They must meet the needs of patients who want the best care possible. Education and research are the primary foci of the professional schools and, where they exist, research centers (Norlin and Osborn, 1998). Educational activities must be responsive to the needs of students, who have the right to expect the best education they can get; research activities must be responsive to the needs of funders, who expect sound inquiry and utility from the research they support (Heyssel, 1984). Each organization also has its own culture. The faculty at professional schools identify most closely with their own discipline rather than any organization, whereas the hospital tends to place greater value on cooperative institutional efforts (Magill et al., 1998).

Thus, even under routine operating conditions, AHCs face an inherent and continuing tension in managing their enterprise. They must simultaneously run each individual entity and carry out each role with excellence, but must also integrate their various distinct organizations and cultures into a cohesive and smoothly running enterprise that collectively is accountable to meeting societal needs. As described throughout this report, however, AHCs are not facing routine operating conditions, so their challenges become even more acute. Whereas coordination and cooperation may not be mandatory during times of growth, they become imperative when retrenchment is required (Magill et al., 1998).

None of the committee's recommendations for transforming the AHC roles can be implemented unless the AHCs' organizational components work together more closely than has historically been required. The demands of transforming the roles surpass the capabilities of any individual organizational component. Although each component will have responsibilities for a portion of the changes required, none can accomplish those changes on their own. In addition, the targets of opportunity are so plentiful that it would be impossible to undertake them all. Even the most generous level of resources is likely to be insufficient given the enormous range of potential activities. Whereas the past decades have been an era of growth for AHCs, during which they were able to expand all of their activities, the coming decades will be an era of choices.

Thus, the primary role of the AHC in the process of change is that of integrator across its organizations and roles. Each role of the AHC can be conducted separately (Heyssel, 1984). Health professions education, research, and clinical care are performed by many organizations that have no affiliation with an AHC. Although organizations performing an individual role make important contributions, the unique contribution of AHCs is their ultimate focus on the impact of their work on people, rather than the individual functions. The external incentives in the recommendations of the prior chapter are designed to support such integration by encouraging planning across the AHC organizations and roles.

The committee offers two broad principles for AHCs to adopt as they endeavor to strengthen the level of integration across their diverse organizations. First, each AHC should develop a shared vision based on the interdependence of their roles and organizations. Although each entity of an AHC will still pursue its own unique objectives, each should also work toward achieving common goals across the AHC (Zelman et al., 1999).

One way of developing a shared vision is for AHCs to make a clear commitment to improving health—of populations as well individual patients—by determining how the AHC overall can have an impact on the health of its patients and the populations that rely on it. This commitment should be stated at the highest levels of the AHC and recognized by its clinical and administrative leaders, the individual organizations that are part of the AHC, its governing body, and its parent university. AHCs typically describe themselves as having a three-part mission encompassing their roles in education, research, and patient care. But a commitment to health involves more than carrying out any individual role; the roles are the means for accomplishing a mission. A commitment to health means starting from the perspective of patient and population needs and asking how the AHC roles can be combined and aligned to have an impact on their health. AHCs will appropriately choose different priorities and approaches to this end and will still carry out a diverse set of activities in their various organizations. In addition, the committee recognizes that having an impact on health may happen over an extended period of time. However, the committee believes it is important for each AHC to develop a shared vision that recognizes the interdependent and complementary nature of their roles within an overall context that encompasses a commitment to health.

Second, each AHC should support openness and transparency of information across the enterprise. All parties should have access to performance information about the entire AHC enterprise for sound decision making and resource allocation (The Blue Ridge Academic Health Group, 1998). Because each organization within the AHC has developed and operated with significant independence, information across the AHC is often weak or unavailable. Although it may be possible to assess how each unit is functioning, it is more difficult to understand the accomplishment of common goals. AHCs should be able to answer such questions as the extent to which clinical care subsidizes research and education; what it costs to train a health professional from initial training to readiness for practice; and, looking at the totality of the research done across all of the organizations in the AHC, what the research portfolio is (and should be) relative to chronic care (for example) or what is known about improving quality. A lack of transparency in setting and communicating strategic priorities creates misunderstandings about the need for change and hampers its progress. Capturing the intellectual energy across the AHC and breaking down barriers within the institutions requires an openness and transparency of information that makes it possible to understand the cross-subsidies and interdependencies across the AHC roles, organizations, and populations served.

The committee offers its final three recommendations with these two broad principles in mind. The principles guide the recommendations, but the recommendations are intended to realize the principles.

Utilizing Information and Communications Technology

Information and communications technology is central to all of the roles of AHCs. Basic biomedical research is becoming increasingly reliant on such technology, and emerging areas, such as genomics and proteomics, require manipulation of large amounts of data. Clinical and health services research, central to translating the results of basic research into clinical care, demand such systems for analysis, synthesis, and dissemination of information. Information and communications technology is also becoming central to clinical education as a teaching tool through the use of simulators and interactive learning models and is making it possible for students to learn to practice in care settings that make more extensive use of advanced clinical information and communications systems. Moreover, delivery of services will increasingly rely on interdisciplinary teams that are linked over time and across settings through this technology. They will also provide a tool for more effective surveillance of health at the community-wide level. Finally, information and communications technology is integral to managing complex systems like AHCs, making strategic decisions, and supporting performance and financial accountability within the institution.

> **Recommendation 5: AHCs must make innovation in and implementation of information technology a priority for both managing the enterprise and conducting their integrated teaching, research, and clinical activities.**
>
> a. AHCs should have information systems that span the enterprise for integrated decision making, performance assessment, and financial management.
>
> b. AHCs need to pioneer the use of information systems for clinical purposes and incorporate their use into clinical education and research.

Given the importance of information and communications technology to the ability of AHCs to perform their roles in the future, it is essential that AHCs make the implementation of such systems a high priority. Capital for information technology needs to be as high a priority as capital for new buildings and medical equipment. If resources for the purpose are not sufficient within AHCs, federal and state governments should consider ways to encourage the needed ongoing investments, particularly for those AHCs that face persistent financial difficulties as a result of serving as safety-net institutions in their communities.

A central goal in improving information technology at AHCs is to maximize the capacity and capability for managing the knowledge and information produced within and used by the AHC in conducting its roles. Knowledge management has clear clinical applications, ensuring that staff has access to all the types of information and knowledge needed to conduct their work, *as* they conduct their work (The Blue Ridge Academic Health Group, 2000). These applications include, for example, access to internal and external databases, sharing of best practices, connections with relevant communities and practices, and synthesized updates of developing knowledge, all of which need to be employed by health professionals who are proficient at accessing, applying, and sharing the knowledge in their daily work (and rewarded for doing so). Knowledge management also applies to any knowledge that is useful and/or essential to the proper management of institutions, teams, departments, and interdisciplinary efforts in conducting clinical care, research, and education. AHCs will need to become more aware of and involved in knowledge management given the expanding knowledge base in health, the potential for genomics research to foster individualized care processes, the expectations of more informed and engaged patients, and demands on them for significant improvements in quality and safety.

To date, the use of information technology at AHCs has focused primarily on meeting institutional needs, driven mainly by clinical operations (The Blue Ridge Academic Health Group, 2000). Current use of information technology at AHCs typically collects and organizes data and may streamline certain work processes (such as ordering tests and reporting results). In some cases, information technology may be in place to guide clinical decision-making. This level of information technology is insufficient for addressing the demands of knowledge management. Knowledge management requires organizational strategies designed to convert information systematically into usable knowledge and enable its sharing and application when and where needed (Detmer, 2001).

Information systems do not automatically lead to knowledge management but are a prerequisite for moving toward it. In recommending that AHCs pioneer the use of information and communications systems, the committee intends that the various components of the AHC initiate (or aggressively continue) discussions with each other about these types of issues, and break down the boundaries that inhibit the sharing of information and knowledge across the AHC organizations and roles.

Although some AHCs have been able to make significant progress in developing their information capabilities, rapid progress by all will require the resolution of issues related to confidentiality of data and data standards. The provisions of the Health Insurance Portability and Accountability Act of 1996 are just going into effect at this writing, so its impact on privacy for patients or on the AHC roles (especially in research) remain to be seen. In terms of standards, the committee urges the development of national data standards to facilitate the development of information technology in the health arena and its incorporation into practice. Standards have been developed by private organizations,[1] but a strong federal role is

---

[1] See, for example, Health Level 7 (HL7), one of the largest private-sector standards-setting organizations, focusing on Version 3 standards for data interchange (Institute of Medicine, 2003).

also required to enhance standardization, thereby ensuring interoperability of systems and comparability of data (Institute of Medicine, 2003). Although AHCs can make some progress in this area, the development of standards can ease the implementation and affordability of information systems for AHCs and others.

Establishing and Measuring AHC-wide Goals for Change

Given the magnitude of the changes required by AHCs, it is important that clear goals be set so that progress toward making those changes can be steadily measured. This information will also be of interest to the public, including federal and state policy makers, payers, and patients. AHCs need to be accountable for the public resources they receive, and policy makers need to be accountable for the way public funds are disbursed.

Recommendation 6: Both AHCs and the public should evaluate the progress of AHCs in: (1) redesigning the content and methods of clinical education; (2) developing organizational structures and team approaches in care to improve health; and (3) increasing emphasis on health services, clinical, prevention, and translational research.

a. To aid AHCs in evaluating their progress, the Secretary of Health and Human Services should:

- Identify broad areas of AHC performance (e.g., quality of education programs, financial accountability).
- Establish an advisory group to suggest guidelines for measurement and examples of measures that could be used by AHCs.
- Obtain information from AHCs related to the broad areas of performance and issue a report every 2 years on progress made in transforming the roles, identifying areas of success as well as obstacles encountered.

b. University leaders and/or AHC boards of trustees should establish mechanisms for accountability and transparency that can be used to assess their progress toward meeting the goals established for transforming the roles of AHCs.

To accomplish the recommendations set forth in this report, AHCs will need to establish measurable goals at the level of the overall AHC. AHCs will need to look across their entire enterprise to align programmatic and financial management, understand the flow of funds, and reorient internal planning and financing arrangements to improve coordination across clinical departments and institutions. Individual organizations within an AHC may set their own objectives, but transforming the roles according to the recommendations in the prior chapter will require better coordination across the entire AHC since (as noted previously) it is not possible for any single AHC organizational component to implement the actions required for a given recommendation independently or to examine one role in isolation from the others.

The challenge in initiating action is that AHCs generally have highly complex governance and management structures. For example, an AHC board may have oversight over the medical school but not the nursing school, or it may contract with several affiliated hospitals but not own one. In such instances, the governing body does not necessarily control the actions of its component units. In some cases, there may not be an oversight board for the AHC at all, with governance being structured at the level of each individual organization that comprises the AHC.

AHCs also commonly face a tension-filled relationship with their parent university (Nonnemaker and Griner, 2001). The university often perceives the AHC as overly focused on clinical activities and not very academic, paying high salaries that cannot be sustained under tenure, unpredictable financially, and overly independent. AHCs often perceive the university as unable to make a decision, overburdened with layers of governance, having little health care expertise, and being exceedingly risk-averse. Change at the AHC often outpaces that at the university (Nonnemaker and Griner, 2001). Furthermore, the various organizational relationships have been quite dynamic in recent years. Changes have typically taken one of two forms (Nonnemaker and Griner, 2001): (1) a change in legal status and the creation of a new entity separate from the main university, or (2) reorganization of existing governance structures, usually to give the AHC greater autonomy to increase its competitiveness in the marketplace.

Within the AHC arrangement, clinical departments have traditionally played a strong role. Department chairs raise funds for research, direct budgets, control faculty promotion, design curriculum in the residency programs, direct the undergraduate medical education process, and are the main source of information and communication between the faculty and the administration (Bulger, 1988). There are both historical and pragmatic reasons for this structure. One is that graduate medical education is accredited through the Accreditation Council of Graduate Medical Education, which is highly structured along departmental and divisional lines. Since accreditation of their graduate medical education programs is critical to most AHCs, there is great reluctance to make significant changes in the departmental organization (Snyderman and Saito, 2000). Moreover, department chairs are reluctant to relinquish their decision-making authority out of concern for the quality of their education and research programs. The departmental structure can also be considered a rational response to the rapid rate in the development of specialization and subspecialization in both the basic and the clinical sciences (The Blue Ridge Academic Health Group, 2001). The departmental structure reflects this clinical specialization and the way work actually gets done.

The strong departments structure, however, also has led to what some have called "semiautonomous baronies" (Ebert and Ginzberg, 1988, p. 14) and "independent fiefdoms" (Munson and D'Aunno, 1989, p. 415), making it difficult to build consensus around broad organization-wide goals. Although an organizational structure along departmental lines has historically enabled AHCs to achieve success in their activities in research, education, and patient care, the question remains of whether it is the best structure to meet the needs of the 21st century.

Their organizational complexity poses a serious challenge to AHCs in developing a vision for the overall AHC enterprise. AHCs have traditionally focused on achieving excellence within each role or independent organizational unit (e.g., the hospital, the medical school); they generally have poor information on their core functions and do not set strategic goals for each (Zelman et al., 1999; The Commonwealth Fund Task Force on Academic Health Centers, 2000a). Performance measures that reflect goals for the entire system are often unavailable since the metrics for measuring success have focused on individual units. For example, a clinical department may document that it is running its residency program effectively, but it is more difficult to assess the extent to which the AHC is developing innovative training methods across its education programs (Zelman et al., 1999). While this situation may be sufficient for operational planning, decisions become more strategic when an organization has to make major changes, and require a more systemwide view and coordination (Zelman et al., 1999).

Two efforts are aimed at helping AHCs improve their understanding of AHC-wide performance. Mission-based management is a measurement and reporting system for understanding the education, research, and patient care activities, although it is focused mainly on the medical school rather than the overall AHC (Association of American Medical Colleges). The primary purpose of mission-based management is as a management tool to integrate the medical school's financial statements, measure and track faculty and departmental activities and contributions, clarify standards for accountability and expectations on overall performance, build organizational support for reporting tools and metrics, guide leadership with dependable data to engage faculty in decision making, hold faculty and department and institutional leaders accountable for performance, and build an institutional perspective. It is not known how widely mission-based approaches have been implemented (Dobson et al., 2002).

Another initiative is the Funds Flow Project of the University

HealthSystem Consortium. This project is designed to provide an understanding of the types and extent of financial transactions that occur across the various enterprises within an AHC, and the economic interrelationships among education, research, and patient care (University HealthSystem Consortium, 2000). The aim is to improve management and business decisions by obtaining a comprehensive financial picture of the entire AHC enterprise. Continuing work will focus on the development of methods for benchmarking so AHCs can have information to compare their performance against that of others. The Blue Ridge Academic Health Group (1998a) has also identified potential performance measures for each role of AHCs, categorizing the measures along four dimensions: productivity, quality, innovation, and societal value. Examples are illustrated in Box 8-1. The groups note that measures related to productivity are more developed than measures in the other categories.

Because of the functional and organizational variability across AHCs, the committee believes that each AHC will need to determine its own goals and priorities and identify specific mechanisms and measures for monitoring their achievement. In recent years, performance measurement has moved toward the use of more standardized measures because they make it pos-

---

BOX 8-1
Examples of AHC Performance Measures from the Blue Ridge Academic Health Group (1998a)

	Productivity	Quality	Innovation	Societal Value
Patient Care	Cost per case	Health-related outcomes	Savings from new clinical protocols	Improvements in community health markers
Research	Direct grant revenue per faculty full-time equivalent (FTE)	Publications per faculty FTE	Reduction in grant preparation time	Cost impact of new diagnostic or treatment capabilities
Education	Contact hours per faculty FTE in teaching	Percentage of students who pass boards	Improvements in student satisfaction or board scores from curricular reforms	Percentage of students who enter primary care or other needed disciplines

sible to draw comparisons, learn from best performers, and identify general areas for improvement (Institute of Medicine, 2002a). However, most current efforts in health focus on clinical care in specific settings, such as hospitals, nursing homes, or home health agencies. For example, a recently announced effort by the Association of American Medical Colleges, the American Hospital Association, and the Federation of American Hospitals is aimed at establishing quality measures for hospital patient care (Association of American Medical Colleges, 2002). Such efforts should have applicability for AHCs but are not sufficient for understanding progress across the AHC roles.

The committee sees applicability in the general approach taken in the Government Performance and Results Act (GPRA). The goal of this legislation, passed in 1993, is to focus on the actual results of government activity and services. Rather than measuring the outputs of an agency, such as grants disbursed or inspections made, GPRA forces agencies to focus on the desired results, such as gains in employment, safety, or quality, and to measure accomplishment of those results (U.S. General Accounting Office, 2002). For example, the goals of the Veterans Administration have included reducing health care costs per patient by 13 percent in 1 year and improving quality as measured by the Chronic Disease Index (U.S. General Accounting Office, 2000). Federal agencies develop their own goals and strategic plans and identify how results will be measured. Because of the diversity of federal agencies, a single set of indicators would not be meaningful, but it was deemed important that each agency set goals specific to its functions and mission, and that the agency be held accountable for achieving those explicitly-stated goals. This is not a simple task and agencies face serious challenges in effecting this level of accountability, including complexities in negotiating across agencies for cross-cutting programs, linking activities and budgets to results, and building the information capacity to meet the demands of GPRA.

In applying this approach to AHCs, the committee recommends that each AHC set and monitor its own measurable goals for transforming each of its roles. Goal setting and strategic planning should occur through clearly established mechanisms that link the organizations in the AHC at the governance, management, and strategic levels. Decision structures need to enable joint problem solving and resolution of the conflicts that are natural and inherent among the AHC's organizations and roles. Despite their interdependence, mechanisms are not always in place to bring the various parties to the table. Although management and governance at each individual organization ensure that its own activities are carried out well, this does not automatically translate into compatible goals across the AHC and may suboptimize priority setting for the AHC overall (for example, decisions about the purchase of medical technology versus information technology, or decisions about space allocations).

Barriers within the AHC need to be broken down to provide opportunities for discussion and decision making by the various interests across the AHC. Some AHCs may do this by tapping into existing interdisciplinary councils or forming new ones to expand the core membership beyond the hospital and medical school. Some may reorganize the flow of information and funds to empower leaders with greater authority to influence and direct change. Some may fundamentally restructure to consolidate governance and management. In one example, the University of California, San Francisco, reorganized to overlay on the departmental structure a research and training organization that would easily let faculty and students cross departmental boundaries to pursue collaborative work. This was accomplished by (1) establishing an executive committee made up of basic science chairs and elected faculty members; (2) centralizing responsibilities for faculty recruitment, admissions, curricula, and facilities with the executive committee; (3) retaining department control over their full-time employees, space, appointments, and promotions; and (4) having each department house one or more research programs so that interdisciplinary research and training programs are administered by individual departments as a resource for all departments (The Blue Ridge Academic Health Group, 2001). In another example, the University of Pennsylvania streamlined its governance by creating a new corporate structure that created a unified governance structure for the school of medicine and clinical components of the AHC, and reduced the number of layers between the university and the individual clinical and academic components of the AHC to three layers from seven (Rodin, 2002). Regardless of the approach taken, the aim is to provide the means and structures for the right players to be at the table, with the right information, from throughout the AHC.

The Secretary of Health and Human Services should support measurement efforts by identifying key dimensions of performance and sample measures for each. This work should be done with input from AHCs, states, and groups that rely on the work of AHCs (e.g., employers that hire their trainees) and should be designed to be useful at both the federal and state levels.

Leadership for Strategic Change Throughout the AHC

The demand for leadership at AHCs has never been greater. In stable times, organizations need good managers, but in times of turmoil and instability, they need strong leadership. If AHC leaders are unable to create a vision for the future and take their organizations forward, AHCs will not succeed, regardless of the support they receive. Society has placed great trust in AHCs to carry out their roles in a way that meets its needs. As society's needs change, so, too, must AHCs.

Recommendation 7: AHCs must be leaders and must develop leaders, at all levels, who can:

a. Manage the organizational and systems changes necessary to improve health through innovation in health professions education, patient care, and research.

b. Improve integration and foster cooperation within and across the AHC enterprise.

c. Improve health by providing guidance on pressing societal problems, such as reduction of health disparities, responses to bioterrorism, or ethical issues that arise in health care, research, and education.

Meeting the strategic challenges set forth in this report will require leadership and innovation at all levels of the AHC. A major role of leadership is to guide organizations in adapting to changing circumstances (Kotter, 1996). Leaders define the future, align people with a vision, and remove obstacles to allow people to realize the vision. Several models describe how organizations undertake major strategic change. While the scope of the present discussion does not permit a comprehensive review, three approaches are briefly described.

Kotter (1996) describes a multistage process designed to overcome the inertia that typically stalls innovation. This eight-step process of change involves: (1) creating a sense of urgency, (2) building the team to lead change, (3) developing a clear vision and strategy, (4) communicating this vision and strategy at every opportunity, (5) eliminating obstacles to action, (6) achieving short-terms wins to create momentum, (7) continuing to make changes, and (8) embedding the changes made in the culture. The first four steps are designed to interrupt the status quo; steps 5 through 7 are designed to introduce new practices; and step 8 is intended to make the changes stick. Although multiple steps may be under way at the same time, they are generally believed to follow this order. Many organizations try to initiate change at step 5 and hit a wall of resistance because of a sense of complacency and a lack of understanding of the need for the change or its course. Although many people believe that initiating change requires a cultural transformation, this framework suggests that cultural change comes at the end of the process, after people's behaviors have changed, and there is a connection between the new actions and improved performance. The new behaviors shape the culture, rather than the reverse.

Another model that has received attention in recent years is the balanced scorecard approach (Kaplan and Norton, 1996), a strategic management system that helps an organization translate its mission and strategy into a set of performance measures to manage the business and build long-term capabilities critical for success. An organization's performance is evaluated along four dimensions: financial performance, customer satisfaction and support, internal processes at which the company must excel, and innovation and learning to constantly improve. The scorecard is balanced in that it considers short- and long-term performance, financial and nonfinancial performance, and internal and external performance, and uses both lagging and leading indicators. Although the process results in a balanced set of performance measures, its aim is to clarify the vision or strategy of top leaders and translate that strategy into operational terms, focusing the entire organization on making the changes that will ensure future success, rather than simply documenting past performance.

The above approaches suggest that strategic change occurs through a linear process. An alternative perspective is provided by theories of complex adaptive systems (Plsek, 2001). A complex adaptive system is a "collection of individual agents that have the freedom to act in ways that are not always predictable and whose actions are interconnected such that one agent's actions changes the context for other agents" (Institute of Medicine, 2001b, p. 312). The actions and reactions of mechanical systems can be well understood, and production can be planned and predicted in great detail. In contrast, in adaptive systems, the parts have the freedom and ability to respond in different ways, with the potential for creativity and innovation (as well as surprises).

Research on complex adaptive systems reveals that relatively few simple rules can guide very complex behaviors and create the conditions for self-organization (Plsek, 2001). For example, the credit card company VISA is based on a few simple rules, such as agreement among banks on card numbering, card appearance, and electronic interface standards. Simple rules tend to fall into three categories: (1) general direction (e.g., leadership aims); (2) prohibitions (e.g., setting boundaries); and (3) provision of resources or permission (e.g., incentives). The theory of complex adaptive systems suggests that fewer (rather than more) rules from leadership can provide a framework for redesign. An AHC can be considered a complex adaptive system in that it has many interrelated parts, but the parts have significant freedom. Although not derived from theories of complex adaptive systems, the beginning of this chapter suggested two simple rules for strategic change in AHCs: commit to health, and ensure transparency of information.

Regardless of whether these or other approaches are taken, all emphasize the importance of a clear aim or vision. A clear and shared vision serves multiple objectives for an AHC. It communicates to internal staff why the organization exists and motivates them around a common good (The Blue Ridge Academic Health Group, 2000a). It helps in the recruitment of personnel whose values are compatible with those of the organization. For audiences outside the AHC, the vision communicates the institution's goals and values. To the extent that the input of external stakeholders is gathered in formulating or affirming a vision, an opportunity is provided to garner external support for the AHC. During times of major change, an enduring vision enables leadership and staff to stay focused on a clear and consistently stated mission (Simone, 1999) and allows leaders to make strategic decisions that are understood by staff and external supporters. Shortell (2002) notes that undertaking strategic change absent a vision is likely to fail because of a lack of understanding of the need for change or the direction of that change. Notes Shortell, if there is no vision, the result is confusion.

Despite the tension common between an AHC and its parent university (noted earlier) university leadership also has a role in supporting the AHC vision and fostering accountability. At one of the meetings of this committee, Judith Rodin, president, University of Pennsylvania, spoke about the challenges that faced the university when its AHC encountered severe financial difficulties. It was perceived that the AHC had pursued an aggressive growth strategy even though its surrounding environment was shifting, and that it had grown beyond its core mission and its capacity. During 1998 and 1999, the AHC lost approximately $300 million, but by 2001 it had a positive bottom line of about $25 million on just its clinical services. This turnaround was achieved through aggressive and decisive leadership from both the university and the AHC and included a complete restructuring and streamlining of governance structures, turnover in senior management staff to bring in leaders who had both the will and the skills to make the needed changes, and strict financial discipline and accountability.

Leadership development involves more than hiring the right person; it needs to be approached as a core system. AHCs have done little in a formal sense to prepare young people for leadership roles or for succession to senior positions. In comments to the committee, Robert Galvin of General Electric estimated that about half of that company's senior management time is devoted to recruiting, developing, and retaining managerial leadership (Galvin, 2002). Four characteristics are reinforced through all levels of the organization and direct how its core leadership is identified and developed: a rigorous financial approach, operational excellence that is value driven and measured constantly, rewards based on performance, and fostering of a team orientation that focuses on the success of the entire company. The core leadership development sequence at General Electric consists of four stages (in order): skill competency, mastery in a field of expertise, development of functional leadership skills, and development of business leadership skills.

The traditional path to AHC leadership is through academic or clinical achievement, although the characteristics required for organizational leadership do not always correlate with the criteria for academic promotions (The Commonwealth Fund Task Force on Academic Health Centers, 2000a). Leading an AHC requires skills in collaboration and teamwork (The Blue Ridge Academic Health Group, 2000a). Management skills, interpersonal skills, and experience are often undervalued, as is the importance of attitude and team compatibility (Simone, 1999). Individual achievement is emphasized. One study of 22 medical school deans found that faculty had been promoted on the basis of individual achievement and that the commitment to collective goals had generally not been rewarded. The Commonwealth Fund Task Force on Academic Health Centers (2000a) also determined that incentives for clinical faculty were not always aligned with the interests of the clinical enterprise. Faculty were often hired with little explicit direction in writing on how they would spend their time, making it difficult to set and enforce expectations for their involvement in patient care, teaching, research, or administration.

The leadership team is also critical in implementing major change. Although leadership may start with one or two people, it needs to grow throughout the organization over time if change is to be sustained (Kotter, 1996). A team is needed to convey needed changes to many constituents and to bring forward the various areas of expertise required for most complex decisions. The membership of the team also matters. If an AHC's leadership team consists of the chief executive officer, chief financial officer, and chief medical officer, the largest segment of the workforce, nurses, is omitted. Such omissions can represent a loss of knowledge to the organization and undermine organizational innovations over time.

Private companies such as General Electric spend years in succession planning and in the development of leaders within the organization, believing that bringing in new leadership from the outside is more often disruptive than successful (The Blue Ridge Academic Health Group, 2001). One estimate suggests that 85 percent of the chief executive officers in private companies are recruited internally (Boufford, 2002). In contrast, AHCs fill the majority of their physician leadership positions through outside recruitment (Schwartz et al., 2000). Although this approach may result in bringing a new and different perspective to bear on the issues confronting the AHC, it may also lead to a lack of continuity in the institution's mission and vision. An existing member of the organization who has been groomed by current leaders can bring a continuity of values and vision, along with knowledge of the organization's culture and characteristics. Midlevel management positions are the training ground for future leaders, where new skills can be practiced. Unfortunately, young people may be discouraged from taking these positions by faculty who regard management as a task for those not able to excel as investigators or clinicians (The Commonwealth Fund Task Force on Academic Health Centers, 2000a).

Leaders in the administrative and managerial aspects of health care delivery also need to improve their use of best evidence for decision making, just as the clinical practice of medicine is expected to rely increasingly on evidence from scientific research. Health care managers generally have been criticized for the overenthusiastic adoption and poor implementation of new business practices and premature discarding of those new initiatives in favor of the latest trend (Walshe and Rundall, 2001). As in evidence-based clinical practice, there are gaps between what is known and what is done, such as slow acceptance of nonphysician practitioners or of community-based treatment options as an alternative to hospitalization. Decision making is based most heavily on operating margins and past budgets (Kovner et al., 2000), an insufficient foundation for the complex decisions faced by AHCs.

Clinical decision making is, by nature, quite different from managerial decision making (Walshe and Rundall, 2001). Clinical decisions tend to be made in a short time frame, and primarily by a single clinician who makes similar types of decisions repeatedly. In contrast, managerial decision making tends to rest more in teams, to have longer time horizons, to be quite varied in its topics, and to face significant constraints on action (e.g., regulations, financing, market competition). Nevertheless, the clear inadequacy of adapting and then discarding managerial initiatives based on little evidence as to their effectiveness argues for the need to develop and utilize an evidence base for management decisions to improve the linkages among research, policy, and practice.

In addition to leading their own organizations, the committee also calls on AHCs to participate in solving the problems society faces in attempting to create healthy populations. This is a much broader perspective than caring for sick people and will require AHCs to work with, educate, and lead their communities in improving health for everybody. Society is facing a number of serious health-related issues, ranging from ethical issues to bioterrorism to end-of-life needs. AHCs need to contribute to the dialogue on these issues and the search for solutions. For example, the Association for Academic Health Centers (2002) has undertaken a major campaign to call attention to the uninsured. Likewise, responding to the threats of bioterrorism will require the involvement of many people and organizations, including AHCs, which can contribute through each of their roles: educating practitioners on proper treatment, conducting research, and caring for patients during an outbreak. AHCs can also work with their local health departments, advise state policy makers on preparedness, and educate community practitioners and the public on appropriate actions.

This report has set forth an agenda for change. As discussed throughout the report, this agenda calls for each AHC role to be adjusted and adapted. Yet accomplishing the necessary transformation for even one role will require enormous energy and leadership and a high level of coordination. And as noted, beyond leading change within their own organizations, AHCs must lead change to improve health for all people. To meet the challenges of the 21st century, AHCs will need public policy support; however, AHCs must also embark on a period of critical self-evaluation and direct the enormous intellectual energy they house toward leading the changes required.

REFERENCES

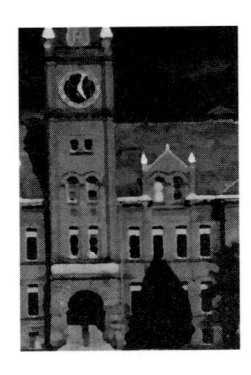

Aaron, H. J., ed. 2001. *The Future of Academic Medical Centers*. Washington, DC: Brookings Institution Press.

AcademyHealth. 2002. *Glossary of Terms Commonly Used in Health Care*. Online. www.academyhealth.org/publications/glossary.htm [accessed February 2002].

Accreditation Council for Graduate Medical Education. 2002. *Principles to Guide the Relationship Between Graduate Medical Education and Industry*. Online. www.acgme.org/New/GMEGuide.pdf.

Accrediting Commission on Education for Health Services Administration. 2001. Online. http://www.acehsa.org/criteria.htm.

Aetna. 2003. *Aetna Announces Initiatives to Reduce the Risks Associated with Racial and Ethnic Disparities in Health*. Online. www.aetna.com/news/2003/prtpr_20030305.htm.

Agency for Healthcare Research and Quality. 2002. *Evidence-based Practice Centers*. Online. www.ahrq.gov/clinic/epc/ [accessed September 2002].

Aiken, L. H. 2001. Evidence-based management: Key to hospital workforce stability. *Journal of Health Administration Education* Spec No:117-124.

———. 2002. Superior outcomes for magnet hospitals: The evidence base. In J. M. McClure and A. S. Hinshaw, eds. *Magnet Hospitals Revisited*. Washington, DC: American Nurses Publishing.

Aiken, L. H., S. Clarke, D. Sloane, J. Sochalski, R. Busse, H. Clarke, P. Giovannetti, J. Hunt, A. M. Rafferty, and J. Shamian. 2001. Nurses' report on hospital care in five countries. *Health Affairs* 20(3):43-53.

American Association of Colleges of Nursing. 2002a. *CCNE: Within Nursing, A Unique Mission*. Online. http://www.aacn.nche.edu [accessed July 9, 2002].

———. 2002b. *Geriatric Nursing Education Project*. Online. www.aacn.nche.edu/Education/Hartford/index.htm.

———. 2002c. *Nursing Faculty Shortage Fact Sheet*. Online. www.aacn.nche.edu/Media/Backgrounders/facultyshortage.htm.

———. 2002d. *Commission on Collegiate Nursing Education Accreditation.* Online. http://www.aacn.nche.edu/Accreditation/index.htm.
American Association of Colleges of Osteopathic Medicine. 2003. *UME-21, Undergraduate Medical Education for the 21st Century: A National Demonstration of Curriculum Innovations to Keep Pace with a Changing Health Care Environment, 1997-2002.* Online. www.aacom.org/ume/.
American Health Care Association. 2002. *AHCA/NCAL Put Forward Long Term Care Financing Reform Proposal.* Online. www.ahca.org/brief/nr020602a.htm [accessed August 14, 2002].
Anderson, G. 2002. *The Roles of Academic Health Centers in the 21st Century: A Workshop Summary.* Washington, DC: The National Academies Press. Online. www.nap.edu/catalog/10383.html.
Anderson, G. F., and J. R. Knickman. 2001. Changing the chronic care system to meet people's needs. *Health Affairs* 20(6):146-160.
Anderson, G. F., E. Steinberg, and R. Heyssel. 1994. The pivotal role of the academic health center. *Health Affairs* 13(3):146-158.
Anderson, G. F., G. Greenberg, and C. K. Lisk. 1999. Academic health centers: Exploring a financial paradox. *Health Affairs* 18(2):156-167.
Anderson, G. F., G. D. Greenberg, and B. O. Wynn. 2001. Graduate medical education: The policy debate. *Annual Review of Public Health* 22:35-147.
Ashton, C. M., N. J. Petersen, J. Souchek, T. J. Menke, H. J. Yu, K. Pietz, M. L. Eigenbrodt, G. Barbour, K. W. Kizer, and N. P. Wray. 1999. Geographic variations in utilization rates in Veterans Affairs hospitals and clinics. *New England Journal of Medicine* 340(1):32-39.
Association of Academic Health Centers. 2002a. *Access to Health Care Initiative.* Online. www.ahcnet.org/programs/delivery/access.php.
———. 2002b. *Frequently Asked Questions.* Online. www.ahcnet.org/newsroom [accessed June 21, 2002].
———. 2002c. *The Nursing Shortage and Academic Health Centers: Assessing Options for Remedy in a Complex System.* Washington, DC: Association of Academic Health Centers.
Association of American Medical Colleges. 1998. *Maximizing the Investment: Principles to Guide the Federal-Academic Partnership in Biomedical and Health Sciences Research.* Washington, DC. Online. www.aamc.org/research/dbr/maximize/contents.htm.
———. 2002. *AAMC Supports National Quality Initiative for Patient Care.* Washington, DC. Online. http://www.aamc.org/newsroom.
———. 2003a. *Columbia University Researchers Receive $6 Million Grant to Establish Health Disparities Center.* Online. www.aamc.org/newsroom/bulletin/columbia/030213.htm.
———. 2003b. *New AAMC Institute to Examine Quality of U.S. Medical Education.* Online. www.aamc.org/newsroom/pressrel/2003/030303.htm.
Association of American Medical Colleges and the Milbank Memorial Fund. 2000. *The Education of Medical Student: Ten Stories of Curriculum Change.* New York, NY: Milbank Memorial Fund.
Association of American Universities. 2000. *Employment Impacts of Academic R&D, Fiscal Year 1999.* Online. www.aau.edu/resuniv/FY97employ.html [accessed February 4, 2002].
Association of Schools of Public Health. 2001. *Annual data report.* Online. www.asph.org.
Barry, M. J., F. J. Fowler Jr., A. G. Mulley Jr., J. V. Henderson Jr., and J. E. Wennberg. 1995. Patient reactions to a program designed to facilitate patient participation in treatment decisions for benign prostatic hyperplasia. *Medical Care* 33(8):771-782.

Barzansky, B., and S. I. Etzel. 2001. Educational programs in U.S. medical schools, 2000-2001. *Journal of the American Medical Association* 286(9):1049-1055.

Batalden, P., D. Leach, S. Swing, H. Dreyfus, and S. Dreyfus. 2002. General competencies and accreditation in graduate medical education. *Health Affairs* 21(5):103-111.

Becher, E. C., and M. R. Chassin. 2001. Improving the quality of health care: Who will lead? *Health Affairs* 20(5):164-179.

Beller, G. A. 2000. President's page: ACC takes strategic steps to address members' needs. American College of Cardiology. *Journal of the American College of Cardiology* 35(7):1989-1992.

Berenson, R. A., and J. Horvath. 2003. Confronting barriers to chronic care management in Medicare. *Health Affairs,* Web Exclusive. Online. www.healthaffairs.org/WebExclusives/2202Berenson.pdf.

Biotechnology Industry Organization. 2003. *Biotechnology: A Collection of Technologies.* Online. www.bio.org/er/technology_collection.asp.

Blendon, R. J., C. Schoen, K. Donelan, R. Osborn, C. M. DesRoches, K. Scoles, K. Davis, K. Binns, and K. Zapert. 2001. Physicians' views on quality of care: A five-country comparison. *Health Affairs* 20(3):233-243.

Blumenthal, D. 1994. The variation phenomenon in 1994. *New England Journal of Medicine* 331(15):1017-1018.

———. 2001. Controlling health care expenditures. *New England Journal of Medicine* 344(10):766-769.

Blumenthal, D., and E. Bass. 2001. The need for data not dogma on the costs of graduate medical education. *Journal of General Internal Medicine* 16(1):66-67.

Blumenthal, D., and M. B. Buntin. 1998. Carve outs: Definition, experience, and choice among candidate conditions. *American Journal of Managed Care* 4(Suppl):SP45-SP57.

Blumenthal, D., and G. S. Meyer. 1996. Academic health centers in a changing environment. *Health Affairs* 15(2):200-215.

Bodenheimer, T., E. H. Wagner, and K. Grumbach. 2002. Improving primary care for patients with chronic illness. *Journal of the American Medical Association* 288(14):1775-1779.

Boufford, J. I. 2002. Leadership and Organizational Change. *Presentation at IOM Annual Meeting.* Online. www.iom.edu/IOM/IOMHome.nsf/Pages/2002+Annual+Meeting+Agenda+leadership.

Bowen, J. L., and D. M. Irby. 2002. Assessing quality and costs of education in the ambulatory setting: A review of the literature. *Academic Medicine* 77(7):621-680.

Boyd, E. A., and L. A. Bero. 2000. Assessing faculty financial relationships with industry: A case study. *Journal of the American Medical Association* 284(17):2209-2214.

Boyle, L. D., and K. Fisher. 2002. *Medicare Direct Graduate Medical Education (DGME) Payments.* Online. www.aamc.org [accessed July 15, 2002].

Broder, S. 2002. *The Roles of Academic Health Centers in the 21st Century: A Workshop Summary.* Washington, DC: The National Academies Press. Online. www.nap.edu/catalog/10383.html.

Brook, R. H. 1997. Managed care is not the problem, quality is. *Journal of the American Medical Association* 278(19):1612-1614.

Brotherton, S. E., F. A. Simon, and S. C. Tomany. 2000. U.S. graduate medical education, 1999-2000. *Journal of the American Medical Association* 284(9):1121-1126.

Bulger, R. J. 1988. Medical education reform and departmental chairs. *Health Affairs* 7(4):185-187.

———. 2000. The quest for the therapeutic organization. *Journal of the American Medical Association* 283(18):2431-2433.

REFERENCES

Bureau of Labor Statistics. 2001. *National Employment and Wage Data from the Occupational Employment Statistical Survey by Occupation.* Online. www.bls.gov/news.release/ocwage.t01.htm [accessed December 8, 2002].

Burton, L. C., J. P. Weiner, G. D. Stevens, and J. Kasper. 2002. Health outcomes and Medicaid costs for frail older individuals: A case study of a MCO versus fee-for-service care. *Journal of the American Geriatrics Society* 50(2):382-388.

Cantor, J. C., A. B. Cohen, D. C. Barker, A. L. Shuster, and R. C. Reynolds. 1991. Medical educators' views on medical education reform. *Journal of the American Medical Association* 26(8):1002-1006.

Cantor, J. C., L. C. Baker, and R. G. Hughes. 1993. Preparedness for practice: Young physicians' views of their professional education. *Journal of the American Medical Association* 270(9):1035-1040.

Cassell, E. J. 1999. Historical perspective of medical residency training: 50 years of changes. *Journal of the American Medical Association* 281(13):1231.

Center for the Evaluative Clinical Sciences at Dartmouth Medical School. 1999a. *Chapter Three—Section 10: Variation Among Regions Served.* Online. http://www.dartmouthatlas.org/99US/toc.php.

———. 1999b. *Chapter Three—Section 13: The Propensity to Hospitalize at Specific Academic Medical Centers.* Online. http://www.dartmouthatlas.org/99US/toc.php.

———. 2003. *About the CECS.* Online. www.dartmouth.edu/dms/cecs/about.html.

Centers for Disease Control and Prevention. 2001. *Center for Chronic Disease Prevention and Health Promotion.* Online. www.cdc.gov/nccdphp/statbook98/background.htm [accessed September 26, 2001].

———. 2002. *Health United States 2002.* Online. www.cdc.gov/nchs/hus.htm.

Centers for Medicare and Medicaid Services. 2003. *HHS to Launch Medicare Demonstrations Projects to Improve Health Care Through Capitated Disease Management Demonstrations.* Online. www.cms.hhs.gov/healthplans/research/CDMPress.pdf.

Chassin, M. R. 1998. Is health care ready for Six Sigma quality? *Milbank Quarterly* 76(4):510, 565-569.

Chassin, M. R., R. W. Galvin, and the Institute of Medicine National Roundtable on Health Care Quality. 1998. The urgent need to improve health care quality. *Journal of the American Medical Association* 280(11):1000-1005.

Christakis, N. A. 1995. The similarity and frequency of proposals to reform U.S. medical education: Constant concerns. *Journal of the American Medical Association* 274(9):706-711.

Christensen, C., R. Bohmer, and J. Kenagy. 2000. Will disruptive innovations cure health care? *Harvard Business Review* September-October:102-112.

Cohen, J. R., and S. Fox. 2003. Developing a new faculty practice plan with a model for funds flow between the hospital and the plan. *Academic Medicine* 78(2):119-124.

Committee on the Roles of Academic Health Centers in the 21st Century. 2002. *The Roles of Academic Health Centers in the 21st Century: A Workshop Summary.* Washington, DC: The National Academies Press. Online. www.nap.edu/catalog/10383.html.

Consumer Reports. 2002. The unraveling of health insurance. *Consumer Reports* 67(7): 48-53.

Conway-Welch, C. 2002. *The Roles of Academic Health Centers in the 21st Century: A Workshop Summary.* Washington, DC: The National Academies Press. Online. www.nap.edu/catalog/10383.html.

Cooper, R. A., T. Henderson, and C. L. Dietrich. 1998. Roles of nonphysician clinicians as autonomous providers of patient care. *Journal of the American Medical Association* 280(9):795-802.

Cooper, R. A., T. E. Getzen, H. J. McKee, and P. Laud. 2002. Economic and demographic trends signal an impending physician shortage. *Health Affairs* 21(1):140-154.

Council on Education for Public Health. 2002. *About Council for Education on Public Health (CEPH).* Online. http://www.ceph.org/about.htm.

Council on Graduate Medical Education (COGME). 2000. *Financing Graduate Medical Education in a Changing Health Care Environment, Fifteenth Report.* Washington, DC: U.S. Department of Health and Human Services, Health Resources and Services Administration.

Crowley, W. F., Jr., and S. O. Thier. 1996. The continuing dilemma in clinical investigation and the future of American health care: A system-wide problem requiring collaborative solutions. *Academic Medicine* 71(11):1154-1163.

Cutler, D. M., and M. McClellan. 2001. Is technological change in medicine worth it? *Health Affairs* 20(5):11-29.

Davies, P., and R. Boruch. 2001. The Campbell Collaboration. *British Medical Journal* (323):294-295.

Davis, K. 2002. *Work in America: Implications for Health Care.* Policy Brief. Council on Health Care Economics and Policy. Online. http://www.sihp.brandeis.edu/council.

DeAngelis, C. D. 2000. The plight of academic health centers. *Journal of the American Medical Association* 283(18):2438-2439.

Detmer, D. E. 1997. Knowledge: A mountain or a stream? *Science* 275:1859.

———. 2001. A new health system and its quality agenda. *Frontiers of Health Services Management* 18(1):3-30.

———. 2003. Building the national health information infrastructure for personal health, health care services, public health and research. *BMC Medical Informatics and Decision Making* 3:1-40. Online. http://www.biomedcentral.com/1472-6947/3/1.

Dobson, A. 2002. *The Roles of Academic Health Centers in the 21st Century: A Workshop Summary.* Washington, DC: The National Academies Press. Online. www.nap.edu/catalog/10383.html.

Dobson, A., L. Koenig, N. Sen, S. Ho, J. Gilani, and The Lewin Group Inc. 2002. *Financial Performance of Academic Health Center Hospitals, 1994-2000.* New York, NY: The Commonwealth Fund.

Doolan, D. F., and D. W. Bates. 2002. Computerized physician order entry systems in hospitals: Mandates and incentives. *Health Affairs* 21(4):180-188.

Dudley, R. A., and H. S. Luft. 2001. Managed care in transition. *New England Journal of Medicine* 344(14):1087-1092.

DukeMed News. 2002. *Duke and Federal Government Partner to Create Innovative Health Care Model.* Online. www.dukemednews.org/global/print.php?context=%2Fnews%2Farticle.php&id=5877.

Eberhardt, D. M. 2001. *Urban and Rural Health Chartbook. Health United States, 2001, Tables 83 and 94.* Online. www.cdc.gov/nchs/hus/htm [accessed July 15, 2002].

Ebert, R. H., and E. Ginzberg. 1988. The reform of medical education. *Health Affairs* 7(2 Suppl):5-38.

Enarson, C., and F. D. Burg. 1992. An overview of reform initiatives in medical education: 1906 through 1992. *Journal of the American Medical Association* 268(9):1141-1143.

Ewan, C. 1985. Curriculum reform: Has it missed its mark? *Medical Education* 19(4):266-275.

Falk, R. H. 2002. Management of atrial fibrillation—radical reform or modest modification? *New England Journal of Medicine* 347(23):1883-1884.

Federation of State Medical Boards. 2002. *State Medical Licensure Requirements and Statistics, 2001-2002.* Online. www.fsmb.org [accessed July 3, 2002].

REFERENCES

Fellows, J. L., A. Trosclair, E. K. Adams, and C. C. Revera. 2002. Annual smoking-attributable mortality, years of potential life lost, and economic costs, United States, 1995-1999. *Journal of the American Medical Association* 287(18):2355-2356.

Fisher, E. S., D. E. Wennberg, T. A. Stukel, D. J. Gottlieb, F. L. Lucas, and E. L. Pinder. 2003. The implications of regional variation in Medicare spending. Part 1: The content quality, and accessibility of care. *Annals of Internal Medicine* 138(4):273-287.

Fontanarosa, P. B., and C. D. DeAngelis. 2002. Basic science and translational research in JAMA. *Journal of the American Medical Association* 287(13):1728.

Foundation for Accountability and The Robert Wood Johnson Foundation. 2002. *A portrait of the chronically ill in America, 2001*. The Robert Wood Johnson Foundation National Strategic Indicator Surveys. Princeton, NJ: The Robert Wood Johnson Foundation.

Fried, B. M., G. C. Weinreich, and K. J. Lester. 2000. E-Health: Technologic revolution meets regulatory constraint. *Health Affairs* 19(6):124-131.

Frist, W. H. 2002. Federal funding for biomedical research: Commitment and benefits. *Journal of the American Medical Association* 287(13):1722-1724.

Gabel, J., L. Levitt, J. Pickreign, H. Whitmore, E. Holve, D. Rowland, K. Dhont, and S. Hawkins. 2001. Job-based health insurance in 2001: Inflation hits double digits, managed care retreats. *Health Affairs* 20(5):180-186.

Galvin, R. 2002. Are AHCs bringing good things to life? Washington, DC: Presentation to Institute of Medicine Committee on the Roles of Academic Health Centers in the 21st Century. July 30.

Garber, A. M. 1994. Can technology assessment control health spending? *Health Affairs* 13(3):115-126.

Gbadebo, A. L., and U. E. Reinhardt. 2001. Economists on academic medicine: Elephants in a porcelain shop? *Health Affairs* 20(2):148-152.

Gelijns, A., and N. Rosenberg. 1994. The dynamics of technological change in medicine. *Health Affairs* 13(3):28-46.

Gelijns, A. C., and S. O. Thier. 2002. Medical innovation and institutional interdependence: Rethinking university-industry connections. *Journal of the American Medical Association* 287(1):72-77.

Gelmon, S. B. 1996. Can educational accreditation drive interdisciplinary learning in the health professions? *Joint Commission Journal on Quality Improvement* 22(3):213-222.

Gelmon, S. B., J. Kimmey, E. O'Neil, and The Task Force on Accreditation of Health Professions Education. 1999. *Strategies for Change and Improvement: The Report of the Task Force on Accreditation of Health Professions Education*. San Francisco, CA: University of California San Francisco, Center for Health Professions.

Ginsburg, P. B. 1999. *Tracking Health Care Costs: Long-Predicted Upturn Appears* (Issue Brief No. 23). Washington, DC: Center for Studying Health System Change.

Goldstein, J. L., and M. S. Brown. 1997. The clinical investigator: Bewitched, bothered and bewildered—but still beloved. *Journal of Clinical Investigation* 99(12):2803-2812.

Goroll, A. H., G. Morrison, E. B. Bass, R. Jablonover, D. Blackman, R. Platt, A. Whelan, and F. P. Hekelman. 2001. Reforming the core clerkship in internal medicine: The SGIM/CDIM Project. Society of General Internal Medicine/Clerkship Directors in Internal Medicine. *Annals of Internal Medicine* 134(1):30-37.

Green, L. A., G. E. Fryer Jr., B. P. Yawn, D. Lanier, and S. M. Dovey. 2001. The ecology of medical care revisited. *New England Journal of Medicine* 344(26):2021-2025.

Greenberg, D. S. 2000. U.S. accelerates investment in biomedical research. *Lancet* 355(9205):731.

Griner, P. F., and D. Danoff. 2000. Sustaining change in medical education. *Journal of the American Medical Association* 283(18):2429-2431.

Grumbach, K. 1999. Primary care in the United States—the best of times, the worst of times. *New England Journal of Medicine* 341(26):2008-2010.
Grumbach, K., and J. Coffman. 1998. Physicians and nonphysician clinicians: Complements or competitors? *Journal of the American Medical Association* 280(9):825-826.
Hanft, R. S. 1988. Thoughts on medical education reform. *Health Affairs* 7(4):187-191.
Hatala, R., and G. Guyatt. 2002. Evaluating the teaching of evidence-based medicine. *Journal of the American Medical Association* 288(9):1110-1112.
Henderson, T. 1999. *Funding of Graduate Medical Education by State Medicaid Programs.* Prepared for the Association of American Medical Colleges, Washington, DC.
———. 2000. *Graduate Medical Education and Public Policy.* 230-00-0089. Washington, DC: U.S. Health Resources and Services Administration.
Heyssel, R. M. 1984. The challenge of governance: The relationship of the teaching hospital to the university. *Journal of Medical Education* 59:162-168.
Hoffman, C., D. Rice, and H. Y. Sung. 1996. Persons with chronic conditions: Their prevalence and costs. *Journal of the American Medical Association* 276:1473-1479.
Holahan, J., and J. Kim. 2000. Why does the number of uninsured Americans continue to grow? *Health Affairs* 19(4):188-196.
Horwitz, R. 2002. *The Roles of Academic Health Centers in the 21st Century: A Workshop Summary.* Washington, DC: The National Academies Press. Online. www.nap.edu/catalog/10383.html.
Hundert, E. 2002. *The Roles of Academic Health Centers in the 21st Century: A Workshop Summary.* Washington, DC: The National Academies Press. Online. www.nap.edu/catalog/10383.html.
Hurley, R., J. Grossman, T. Lake, and L. Casalino. 2002. A longitudinal perspective on health plan-provider risk contracting. *Health Affairs* 21(4):144-153.
Hwang, W., W. Weller, H. Ireys, and G. Anderson. 2001. Out-of-pocket medical spending for care of chronic conditions. *Health Affairs* 20(6):267-278.
Iglehart, J. K. 1994. Rapid changes for academic medical centers. 1. *New England Journal of Medicine* 331(20):1391-1395.
———. 1995. Rapid changes for academic medical centers. 2. *New England Journal of Medicine* 332(6):407-411.
Institute for the Future. 2000. *Health and Health Care 2010: The Forecast, The Challenge.* San Francisco, CA: Jossey-Bass Publishers.
Institute of Medicine. 1994. *Careers in Clinical Research, Obstacles and Opportunities.* Washington, DC: National Academy Press.
———. 1996. *The Nation's Physician Workforce: Options for Balancing Supply and Requirements.* Washington, DC: National Academy Press.
———. 2000. *To Err Is Human: Building a Safer Health System.* Washington, DC: National Academy Press.
———. 2001a. *Preserving Public Trust: Accreditation and Human Research Participant Protections.* Washington, DC: National Academy Press.
———. 2001b. *Coverage Matters: Insurance and Health Care.* Washington, DC: National Academy Press.
———. 2001c. *Crossing the Quality Chasm: A New Health System for the 21st Century.* Washington, DC: National Academy Press.
———. 2002a. *Health Insurance Is a Family Matter.* Washington, DC: The National Academies Press.
———. 2002b. *Leading by Example, Coordinating Government Roles in Improving Health Care Quality.* Washington, DC: The National Academies Press.
———. 2002c. *Responsible Research.* Washington, DC: The National Academies Press.

———. 2002d. *The Role of Purchasers and Payers in the Clinical Research Enterprise: Workshop Summary*. Washington, DC: The National Academies Press.
———. 2003a. *Unequal Treatment: Confronting Racial and Ethnic Disparities in Health Care*. Washington, DC: The National Academies Press.
———. 2003b. *The Future of the Public's Health in the 21st Century*. Washington, DC: The National Academies Press.
———. 2003c. *Fostering Rapid Advances in Health Care, Learning from System Demonstrations*. Washington, DC: The National Academies Press.
———. 2003d. *Health Professions Education: A Bridge to Quality*. Washington, DC: The National Academies Press.
———. 2003e. *Priority Areas for National Action*. Washington, DC: The National Academies Press.
———. 2003f. *Who Will Keep the Public Healthy? Educating Public Health Professionals for the 21st Century*. Washington, DC: The National Academies Press.
Irby, D. M. 1995. Teaching and learning in ambulatory care settings: A thematic review of the literature. *Academic Medicine* 70(10):898-931.
James, B. C. 2001. Making it easy to do it right. *New England Journal of Medicine* 345(13):991-993.
Jonas, H. S., S. I. Etzel, and B. Barzansky. 1990. Undergraduate medical education. *Journal of the American Medical Association* 264(7):801-809.
Josiah Macy, Jr. Foundation. 1999. *Education for More Synergistic Practice of Medicine and Public Health*. New York, NY: Josiah Macy, Jr. Foundation.
Kaiser Family Foundation and Health Research and Educational Trust. 2001. *Employer Health Benefits, 2001 Summary of Findings*. Online. www.kff.org [accessed October 31, 2001].
Kalfoglou, A., and N. S. Sung. 2002. What inspires clinical research trainees and keeps them on the path? *Journal of Investigative Medicine* 50(6):408-411.
Kane, N. M. 2001. The financial health of academic medical centers: An elusive subject. In H. J. Aaron, editor, *The Future of Academic Medical Centers*. Washington, DC: Brookings Institution Press.
Kaplan, R. S., and D. P. Norton. 1996. *Translating Strategy into Action: The Balanced Scorecard*. Boston, MA: Harvard Business School Press.
Kassirer, J. P. 1994. Academic medical centers under siege. *New England Journal of Medicine* 331(20):1370-1371.
———. 1996. Redesigning graduate medical education—location and content. *New England Journal of Medicine* 335(7):507-509.
———. 2000. Patients, physicians, and the Internet. *Health Affairs* 19(6):115-123.
Kaufman, A. 1999. How to teach for more synergistic practice: Didactic, experimental, teaching sites, multiprofessional team teaching, use of information systems. *Education for More Synergistic Practice of Medicine and Public Health*. In M. Hager, ed. New York, NY: Josiah Macy, Jr. Foundation.
Kaufman, A., D. Derksen, S. McKernan, P. Galbraith, S. Sava, J. Wills, and E. Fingado. 2000. Managed care for uninsured patients at an academic health center: A case study. *Academic Medicine* 75(4):323-330.
Kindig, D. A., N. C. Dunham, and J. M. Eisenberg. 1999. Needs and challenges for health services research at academic health centers. *Academic Medicine* 74(11):1193-1201.
Kirch, D. 2002. *The Roles of Academic Health Centers in the 21st Century: A Workshop Summary*. Washington, DC: The National Academies Press. Online. www.nap.edu/catalog/10383.html.
Kleinke, J. D. 2000. Vaporware.com: The failed promise of the health care Internet. *Health Affairs* 19(6):57-71.

Korn, D. 1996. Reengineering academic medical centers: Reengineering academic values? *Academic Medicine* 71(10):1033-1043.

———. 2000. Conflicts of interest in biomedical research. *Journal of the American Medical Association* 184(17):2234-2237.

———. 2002. The NIH budget in the "postdoubling era." *Science* 296:1401-1402.

Kotter, J. 1996. *Leading Change*. Boston, MA: Harvard Business School Press.

Kovner, A. R., J. J. Elton, and J. Billings. 2000. Evidence-based management. *Frontiers of Health Services Management* 16(4):3-24.

Laine, C., and F. Davidoff. 1996. Patient-centered medicine: A professional evolution. *Journal of the American Medical Association* 275(2):152-156.

Larson, E. 2001. Opportunities to improve the relationship between nursing and medicine in practice. *Enhancing Interactions Between Nursing and Medicine*. In M. Hager, ed. New York, NY: Josiah Macy, Jr. Foundation.

Lave, J. R. 2001. Reflections on "a longitudinal study of the effects of graduate medical education on hospital operating costs". *Health Service Research* 35(6):1203-1206.

LeRoy, L. B. 1994. Meeting the challenge: A health workforce prepared for the future. *Inquiry* 31(3):334-337.

Levit, K., C. Smith, C. Cowan, H. Lazenby, A. Sensenig, and A. Catlin. 2003. Trends in U.S. health care spending, 2001. *Health Affairs* 22(1):154-164.

Lewin, L. 2002. *The Roles of Academic Health Centers in the 21st Century: A Workshop Summary*. Washington, DC: The National Academies Press. Online. www.nap.edu/catalog/10383.html.

Ludmerer, K. 1999. *Time to Heal: American Medical Education from the Turn of the Century to the Era of Managed Care*. New York, NY: Oxford University Press.

Lurie, N., and M. B. Buntin. 2002. Health disparities and the quality of ambulatory care. *New England Journal of Medicine* 347(21):1709-1710.

Magill, M. K., P. Catinella, L. Haas, and C. C. Hughes. 1998. Cultures in conflict: A challenge to faculty of academic health centers. *Academic Medicine* 73(8):871-875.

Manning, F. J. 2000. *Summary of the June 2000 Meeting of the Clinical Research Roundtable*. Washington, DC. Online. www.iom.edu/hsp.

Matherlee, K. 1995. The outlook for clinical research: Impacts of federal funding restraint and private sector reconfiguration. *Academic Medicine* 70(12):1065-1072.

———. 2000. *Reshaping AHCs' Role in Biomedical Research*. Issue Brief No. 751. Washington, DC: National Health Policy Forum.

———. 2001. *Federal and State Perspectives on GME Reform*. Issue Brief No. 764. Washington, DC: National Health Policy Forum.

Mays, G. P., R. E. Hurley, and J. M. Grossman. 2001. *Consumers Face Higher Costs As Health Plans Seek to Control Drug Spending* (Issue Brief No. 45). Washington, DC: Center for Studying Health System Change.

McGinnis, M. J., P. Williams-Russo, and J. R. Knickman. 2002. The case for more active policy attention to health promotion. *Health Affairs* 21(2):78-93.

Medicare Payment Advisory Commission (MedPAC). 1999. *Report to Congress: Rethinking Medicare's Payment Policies for Graduate Medical Education and Teaching Hospitals*. Washington, DC: Medicare Payment Advisory Commission.

———. 2001. *Report to Congress: Medicare Payment for Nursing and Allied Health Education*. Washington, DC: Medicare Payment Advisory Commission.

———. 2002. *Section 2B, Hospital Inpatient and Outpatient Services. Report to Congress: Medicare Payment Policy*. Washington, DC: Medicare Payment Advisory Commission.

———. 2003. *Report to Congress: Medicare Payment Policy*. Washington, DC: Medicare Payment Advisory Commission. Online. www.medpac.gov.

Midwest Business Group on Health, Juran Institute, and The Severyn Group Inc. 2002. *Reducing the Costs of Poor-Quality Health Care Through Responsible Purchasing Leadership.* Chicago, IL: Midwest Business Group on Health. Online. www.mbhg.org.

Morin, K., H. Rakatansky, F. A. Riddick Jr., L. J. Morse, J. M. O'Bannon III, M. S. Goldrich, P. Ray, M. Weiss, R. M. Sade, and M. A. Spillman. 2002. Managing conflicts of interest in the conduct of clinical trials. *Journal of the American Medical Association* 287(1):78-84.

Morrissey, J. 2002. Doctor's orders: Computerized decision support system directs Vanderbilt physicians to the latest treatment data, helping to eliminate unnecessary costs. *Modern Healthcare*, April 22.

Moseley, J. B., K. O'Malley, N. J. Petersen, T. J. Menke, B. A. Brody, D. H. Kuykendall, J. C. Hollingsworth, C. M. Ashton, and N. P. Wray. 2002. A controlled trial of arthroscopic surgery for osteoarthritis of the knee. *New England Journal of Medicine* 347(2):81-88.

Moses, H., and J. B. Martin. 2001. Academic relationships with industry. *Journal of the American Medical Association* 285(7):933-935.

Moy, E., P. F. Griner, D. R. Challoner, and D. R. Perry. 2000. Distribution of research awards from the National Institutes of Health among medical schools. *New England Journal of Medicine* 342(4):250-255.

Mukamel, D. B., H. Temkin-Greener, and M. L. Clark. 1998. Stability of disability among PACE enrollees: Financial and programmatic implications. *Health Care Financing Review* 19(3):83-100.

Mundinger, M. O. 2002. Through a different looking glass. *Health Affairs* 21(1):163-164.

Munson, F. C., and T. A. D'Aunno. 1989. Structural change in academic health centers. *Hospital and Health Services Administration* 34(3):413-425.

Myers, C., N. Paulk, and C. Dudlak. 2001. Genomics: Implications for health systems. *Frontiers in Health Services Management* 17(3):3-16.

Nathan, D. G. 1998. Clinical research: Perceptions, reality, and proposed solutions. *Journal of the American Medical Association* 280(16):1427-1431.

———. 2002. Careers in translational clinical research—historical perspectives, future challenges. *Journal of the American Medical Association* 287(18):2424-2427.

National Advisory Council on Nurse Education and Practice. 1996. *Report to the Secretary of the Department of Health and Human Services on the Basic Registered Nurse Workforce.* U.S. Department of Health and Human Services, Bureau of Health Professions, Division of Nursing. Online. ftp://ftp.hrsa.gov/bhpr/nursing/bwreport/BWFull.pdf.

———. 1997. *A National Informatics Agenda for Nursing Education and Practice.* U.S. Department of Health and Human Services, Bureau of Health Professions, Division of Nursing. Online. ftp://ftp.hrsa.gov/bhpr/nursing/nireport/NIFull.pdf.

National Cancer Institute. 2002. *Description of Cancer Centers Program.* Online. www3.cancercenters.gov/cancercenters/description.html.

National Center for Chronic Disease Prevention and Health Promotion. 1999. *About Chronic Disease.* Online. www.cdc.gov/nccdphp.about.htm [accessed September 26, 2001].

National Center for Complementary and Alternative Medicine. 2001. *Expanding Horizons of Health Care, Five Year Strategic Plan 2001-2003.* Online. www.nccam.nih.gov/about/plans/fiveyear/fiveyear.pdf [accessed March 15, 2002].

National Center for Health Statistics. 1999. *Health, United States, 1999. With Health and Aging Chartbook.* Hyattsville, MD: Government Printing Office.

———. 2002. *Health United States, 2002.* Online. www.dcd.gov/nchs [accessed December 10, 2002].

National Heart, Lung and Blood Institute. 2003. *Framingham Heart* Study. Online. www.nhlbi.nih.gov/about/framingham/.

National Institute of Diabetes and Digestive and Kidney Diseases. *Diabetes Control and Complications Trial.* Online. http://www.niddk.nih.gov/health/diabetes/pubs/dcct1/dcct.htm [accessed December 9, 2002].

National Institute of Neurological Disorders and Stroke, ed. 1999. *Neuroscience at the New Millennium.* NIH Publication No. 99-4566. Bethesda, MD: National Institutes of Health.

National Institutes of Health. 1997. *Executive Summary, NIH Director's Panel on Clinical Research Report.* Online. www.nih.gov/news/crp/97report/execsum/htm [accessed October 1, 2002].

―――. 2001. *NIH Support to U.S. Medical Schools, FY's 1970-2000–TOTALS.* http://grants1.nih.gov/grants/award/trends/medsup7000.txt.

―――. 2002a. *Structural Biology at NIH, Overview.* Online. www.nih. gov/sigs/SBC/overview.htm [accessed June 21, 2002].

―――. 2002b. *Award data.* Online. http://grants1.nih.gov/grants/awards/trends/compaw1.htm.

―――. 2003. Summary of the FY 2004 President's Budget. Washington, DC: National Institutes of Health. Online. www.nih.gov/news/budgetfy2004/fy2004presidentsbudget.pdf.

National Institutes of Health Bioengineering Consortium. 1997. NIH working definition of bioengineering. Online. www.beacon1.nih.gov/bioengineering_definition.htm [accessed June 2002].

National League for Nursing Accreditation Commission. 2001. Council for higher education accreditation (CHEA) recognition of NLAC. Online. http://www.nlnac.org/about%20NLNAC/chea_recognition_of_nlnac.htm.

National Research Council. 2000. *Addressing the Nation's Changing Needs for Biomedical and Behavioral Scientists.* Washington, DC: National Academy Press.

National Science and Technology Council. 2000. *Discovery, Education and Innovation: An Overview of the Federal Investment in Science and Technology.* Online. www.ostp.gov/NSTC/html/dei/index/html [accessed November 21, 2002].

Neumann, P. J., and E. A. Sandberg. 1998. Trends in health care R&D and technology innovation. *Health Affairs* 17(6):111-119.

Newhouse, J. P., and G. R. Wilensky. 2001. Paying for graduate medical education: The debate goes on. *Health Affairs* 20(2):136-147.

Nonnemaker, L., and P. F. Griner. 2001. The effects of a changing environment on relationships between medical schools and their parent universities. *Academic Medicine* 76(1):9-18.

Norlin, C., and L. M. Osborn. 1998. Organizational responses to managed care: Issues for academic health centers and implications for pediatric programs. *Pediatrics* 101(4):805-812.

O'Connor, G. T., H. B. Quinton, N. D. Traven, L. D. Ramunno, T. A. Dodds, T. A. Marciniak, and J. E. Wennberg. 1999. Geographic variation in the treatment of acute myocardial infarction: The Cooperative Cardiovascular Project. *Journal of the American Medical Association* 281(7):627-633.

Office of Extramural Research. 2002. *Imaging at the Molecular and Cellular Levels.* Online. http://grnats1.nih.gov/grants/bioimaging/molecular.htm [accessed June 2002].

Oinonen, M. J., W. F. Crowley Jr., J. Moskowitz, and P. H. Vlasses. 2001. How do academic health centers value and encourage clinical research? *Academic Medicine* 76(7):700-706.

Osterweis, M. 1999. The evolving structure, organization and governance of academic health centers. Chapter 2 in *Mission Management, A New Synthesis, Volume 1.* R. Bulger, M. Osterweis, and E. Rubin, eds. Washington, DC: Association of Academic Health Centers.

_____. 2001. Collaborative models—what is working well? *Enhancing Interactions Between Nursing and Medicine.* In M. Hager, ed. New York, NY: Josiah Macy, Jr. Foundation.

Petersdorf, R. G., and K. S. Turner. 1995. Medical education in the 1990s—and beyond: A view from the United States. *Academic Medicine* 70(7 Suppl):S41-47, discussion S48-S50.

Pew Health Professions Commission. 1998. *Beyond the Balanced Budget Act of 1997: Strengthening Federal GME Policy.* Online. www.futurehealth.ucsf.edu/publications/publications_archive.html.

Pharmaceutical Research and Manufacturers of America (PhRMA). 2002. *PhRMA Industry Profile 2001.* Online. www.phrma.org/publications/publications/profile02/index.cfm.

Phillips, R. L., D. C. Harper, M. Wakefield, L. A. Green, G. E. Freyer Jr. 2002. Can nurse practitioners and physicians beat parochialism into plowshares? *Health Affairs* 21(5):133-142.

Plsek, P. 2001. Redesigning health care with insights from the science of complex adaptive systems. Appendix B in *Crossing the Quality Chasm, A New Health System for the 21st Century.* Washington, DC: National Academy Press.

Pober, J. S., C. S. Neuhauser, and J. M. Pober. 2001. Obstacles facing translational research in academic medical centers. *FASEB Journal* 15(13):2303-2313.

Pollard, T. D. 2002. The future of biomedical research: From the inventory of genes to understanding physiology and the molecular basis of disease. *Journal of the American Medical Association* 287(13):1725-1727.

Program of All Inclusive Care for the Elderly. 2002. Online. www.natlpaceassn.org [accessed December 7, 2002].

Regan-Smith, M. G. 1998. Reform without change: Update, 1998. *Academic Medicine* 73(5):505-507.

Rettig, R. A. 2000. The industrialization of clinical research. *Health Affairs* 19(2):129-146.

Reuter, J. 1999. *Patterns of Specialty Care: Academic Health Centers and the Patient Care Mission.* New York, NY: The Commonwealth Fund.

Reynolds, C. F., III, S. Adler, S. L. Kanter, J. P. Horn, J. Harvey, and G. M. Bernier Jr. 1995. The undergraduate medical curriculum: Centralized versus departmentalized. *Academic Medicine* 70(8):671-675.

Rimar, S. 2000. Strategic planning and the balanced scorecard for faculty practice plans. *Academic Medicine* 75(12):1186-1188.

Robertson, J. A., B. Brody, A. Buchanan, J. Kahn, and E. McPherson. 2002. Pharmacogenetic challenges for the health care system. *Health Affairs* 21(4):155-167.

Robinson, J. C. 2002. "Renewed emphasis on consumer cost sharing in health insurance benefit design." Health Affairs Web Exclusive. Online. www.healthaffairs.org/webexclusives/robinson_web_excl_032002.htm [accessed April 4, 2002].

_____. 2003. Hospital tiers in health insurance: Balancing consumer choice with financial institutions. *Health Affairs* Web Exclusive. Online. www.healthaffairs.org/WebExclusives/CHCF_Web_Excl_031903.htm.

Rodin, J. 2002. The Future of Academic Health Centers in America. Washington, DC: Presentation to Institute of Medicine Committee on the Roles of Academic Health Centers in the 21st Century, April 17.

Rosenberg, C. 1987. *The Care of Strangers: The Rise of America's Hospital System.* New York, NY: Basic Books.

Rundall, T. G., S. M. Shortell, M. C. Wang, L. Casalino, T. Bodenheimer, R. R. Gillies, J. A. Schmittdiel, N. Oswald, and J. C. Robinson. 2002. As good as it gets? Chronic care management in nine leading U.S. physician organisations. *British Medical Journal* 325(7370):958-961.

Sachdeva, A. K. 2000. Faculty development and support needed to integrate the learning of prevention in the curricula of medical schools. *Academic Medicine* 75(7 Suppl):S35-S42.

Safriet, B. J. 1994. Impediments to Progress in Health Care Workforce Policy: License and Practice Laws. *Inquiry* 31(3):310-317.

Salinksy, E. 2002. *Will the Nation Be Ready for the Next Bioterrorism Attack? Mending Gaps in the Public Health Infrastructure.* NHPF Issue Brief No. 776. Washington, DC: National Health Policy Forum.

Salsberg, E. 2001. *Dilemmas Around the Junior Workforce and Indentured Service/Apprenticeship Model for Graduate Medical Education in the USA.* Fifth International Physician Workforce Conference, Sydney, Australia. Online. http://chws.albany.edu/reports/022001/dilgme2001.pdf.

Samuels, S. 2001. The economics of genomics. *Frontiers of Health Services Management* 17(3):35-38, discussion 39-44.

Samuelson, P. A. and W. D. Nordhaus. 1989. *Economics.* New York, NY: McGraw-Hill.

Schechter, A. N. 1998. The crisis in clinical research: Endangering the half-century National Institutes of Health Consensus. *Journal of the American Medical Association* 280(16):1440-1442.

Schneider, E., and J. M. Eisenberg. 1998. Strategies and methods for aligning current and best medical practices. *Western Journal of Medicine* 168(5):311-318.

Schneider, S. 2002. Information therapy answers the Institute of Medicine's harsh report. *Managed Care Quarterly* 10(1):7-10.

Schoen, C., R. J. Blendon, C. M. DesRoches, and R. Osborn. 2002. *Comparison of Health Care System Views and Experience in Five Nations, 2001.* New York, NY: The Commonwealth Fund.

Schroeder, S. A., J. S. Zones, and J. A. Showstack. 1989. Academic medicine as a public trust. *Journal of the American Medical Association* 262(6):803-812.

Schwartz, R. W., C. R. Pogge, S. A. Gillis, and J. W. Holsinger. 2000. Programs for the development of physician leaders: A curricular process in its infancy. *Academic Medicine* 75(2):133-140.

Shortell, S. 2002. *Effective Organizational Change: Assessing the Evidence. Presentation at IOM Annual Meeting.* Online. www.iom.edu/IOM/IOMHome.nsf/Pages/2002+Annual+Meeting+Agenda+leadership.

Showstack, J. 1999. Interdisciplinary education in a specialized society. *Education for More Synergistic Practice of Medicine and Public Health.* In M. Hager, ed. New York, NY: Josiah Macy, Jr. Foundation.

Shuster, M., E. McGlynn, and R. Brook. 1996. How good is the quality of health care in the United States? *Milbank Quarterly* 76(4):517-563.

Simone, J. V. 1999. Understanding academic medical centers: Simone's maxims. *Clinical Cancer Research* 5(9):2281-2285.

Snyderman, R. 2002. *The Roles of Academic Health Centers in the 21st Century: A Workshop Summary.* Washington, DC: The National Academies Press. Online. www.nap.edu/catalog/10383.html.

Snyderman, R., and V. Y. Saito. 2000. *Academic Health Systems in Transition, 2000.* Chapel Hill, NC: Duke University Medical Center and Health System.

Snyderman, R., G. F. Sheldon, and T. A. Bishcoff. 2002. Gauging supply and demand: The challenging quest to predict the future physician workforce. *Health Affairs* 21(1):167-168.

Sochalski, J., L. H. Aiken, and C. M. Fagin. 1997. Hospital restructuring in the United States, Canada, and Western Europe: An outcomes research agenda. *Medical Care* 35(10 Suppl):OS13-OS25.

Social Security Administration and Medicare Boards of Trustees. 2002. *Status of the Social Security and Medicare Programs: A Summary of the 2002 Annual Reports*. Washington, DC: Social Security Administration. Online. www.ssa.gov/OACT/TRSUM/trsummary.html.
Starr, P. 2000. Health care reform and the new economy. *Health Affairs* 19(6):23-32.
Steinbrook, R. 2002. Nursing in the crossfire. *New England Journal of Medicine* 346(22):1757-1766.
Strunk, B., and P. Ginsburg. 2002. *Aging Plays a Limited Role in Health Care Cost Trends*. (Data Bulletin No. 23). Washington, DC: Center for Studying Health System Change.
Strunk, B. C., P. B. Ginsberg, and J. R. Gabel. 2001. *Tracking Health Care Costs: Hospital Care Key Cost Driver in 2002*. (Data Bulletin No. 21- Revised). Washington, DC: Center for Studying Health System Change.
Stryer, D., S. Tunis, H. Hubbard, and C. Clancy. 2000. The outcomes of outcomes and effectiveness research: Impacts and lessons from the first decade. *Health Services Research* 35(5)Pt 1:977-993.
Sung, N. S., W. F. Crowley, M. Genel, P. Salber, L. Sandy, L. Sherwood, S. Johnson, V. Catanese, H. Tilson, K. Getz, E. Larson, D. Scheinberg, A. Reece, H. Slavkin, A. Dobs, J. Grebb, R. Martinez, A. Korn, and D. Rimoin. 2003. Central challenges facing the national clinical research enterprise. *Journal of American Medical Association* 289(10):1278-1287.
The Blue Ridge Academic Health Group. 1998a. *Report 1: Academic Health Centers: Getting Down to Business*. Charlottesville, VA: University of Virginia.
———. 1998b. *Report 2: Promoting Value and Expanded Coverage: Good Health Is Good Business*. Charlottesville, VA: University of Virginia.
———. 2000a. *Report 3: Into the 21st Century: Academic Health Centers as Knowledge Managers*. Charlottesville, VA: University of Virginia.
———. 2000b. *Report 4: In Pursuit of Greater Value: Stronger Leadership in and by Academic Health Centers*. Charlottesville, VA: University of Virginia.
———. 2001. *Report 6: Creating a Value-Driven Culture and Organization in the Academic Health Center*. Charlottesville, VA: University of Virginia.
The Commonwealth Fund Task Force on Academic Health Centers. 1997a. *Understanding the Social Mission of Academic Health Centers*. New York, NY: The Commonwealth Fund.
———. 1997b. *Leveling the Playing Field: Financing the Mission of Academic Health Centers*. New York, NY: The Commonwealth Fund.
———. 1999. *From Bench to Bedside*. New York, NY: The Commonwealth Fund.
———. 2000a. *Health Care at the Cutting Edge: The Role of Academic Health Centers in the Provision of Specialty Care*. New York, NY: The Commonwealth Fund.
———. 2000b. *Managing Academic Health Centers: Meeting the Challenges of the New Health Care World*. New York, NY: The Commonwealth Fund.
———. 2001. *Shared Responsibility: Academic Health Centers and the Provision of Care to the Poor and Uninsured*. New York, NY: The Commonwealth Fund.
———. 2002. *Training Tomorrow's Doctors*. New York, NY: The Commonwealth Fund.
The Kaiser Family Foundation. 2001. *Safety Net Hospital Responses*. Online. http://www.kff.org [accessed December 7, 2002].
The Robert Wood Johnson Foundation. 1996. *Chronic Care in America: A 21st Century Challenge*. Princeton, NJ: The Robert Wood Johnson Foundation.
Thier, S. O. 1994. Academic medicine's choices in an era of reform. *Academic Medicine* 6(3):185-189.
University of California, 2003. *UC Unveils Pioneering Web-Based Medical-Event Reporting System*. Online. www.ucop.edu/news/archives/2003/mar27art1.html.

University of Cincinnati Medical Center. 2002. *University of Cincinnati Medical Center Economic Impact Study, Executive Summary*. Online. www.medcenter.uc.edu/impact/cfm [accessed May 1, 2002].
University of Virginia Health System. 2003. *Health Evaluation Sciences*. Online. hesweb1.med.virginia.edu/HES_background.htm.
U.S. General Accounting Office. 2000. *Managing for Results: Continuing Challenges to Effective GPRA Implementation*. GAO/T-GGD-00-178.
———. 2001. *Biomedical Research: HHS Direction Needed to Address Financial Conflicts of Interest*. GAO-02-89. Washington, DC: US General Accounting Office.
———. 2002. *Reports on the Government Performance and Results Act*. Online. http://www.gao.gov/new.items/gpra/gpra.htm [accessed April 4, 2003].
Vaitukaitis, J. L. 2000. Reviving patient-oriented research. *Academic Medicine* 75(7):683-685.
Vladeck, B. 2002. *The Roles of Academic Health Centers in the 21st Century: A Workshop Summary*. Washington, DC: The National Academies Press. Online. www.nap.edu/catalog/10383.html.
Wagner, E. H., P. Barrett, M. J. Barry, W. Barlow, and F. J. Fowler Jr. 1995. The effect of a shared decisionmaking program on rates of surgery for benign prostatic hyperplasia. Pilot results. *Medical Care* 33(8):765-770.
Wagner, E. H., B. T. Austin, and M. Von Korff. 1996. Improving outcomes in chronic illness. *Managed Care Quarterly* 4(2):12-25.
Wagner, E. H., B. T. Austin, C. Davis, M. Hindmarsh, J. Schaefer, and A. Bonomi. 2001. Improving chronic illness care: Translating evidence into action. *Health Affairs* 20(6):64-78.
Walshe, K., and T. G. Rundall. 2001. Evidence-based management: From theory to practice in health care. *Milbank Quarterly* 79(3):429-458.
Walston, S. L., L. R. Burns, and J. R. Kimberly. 2000. Does reengineering really work? An examination of the context and outcomes of hospital reengineering initiatives. *Health Services Research* 34(6):1363-1388.
Waxman, H. S., and H. R. Kimball. 1999. Assessing continuing medical education. *American Journal of Medicine* 107(1):1-4.
Weed, L. L. 1981. Physician of the future. *New England Journal of Medicine* 304(15):903-907.
Weed, L. L., and L. Weed. 1999. Opening the black box of clinical judgment—an overview. *British Medical Journal* 319(7220):1279.
Weisbrod, B. A., and C. L. LaMay. 1999. Mixed signals: Public policy and the future of health care R&D. *Health Affairs* 18(2):112-125.
Weissman, J. S., D. Saglam, E. G. Campbell, N. Causino, and D. Blumenthal. 1999. Market forces and unsponsored research in academic health centers. *Journal of the American Medical Association* 281(12):1093-1098.
Welch, H. G., and J. D. Lurie. 2000. Teaching evidence-based medicine: Caveats and challenges. *Academic Medicine* 75(3):235-240.
Wennberg, J. E. 1999. Understanding geographic variations in health care delivery. *New England Journal of Medicine* 340(1):52-53.
———. 2002. Unwarranted variations in healthcare delivery: Implications for academic medical centres. *British Medical Journal* 325(7370):961-964.
Wennberg, J., E. Fisher, and J. Skinner. 2002. *Geography Debate over Medicare Reform*. Online. www.healthaffairs.org [accessed February 13, 2002].

Wieland, D., V. L. Lamb, S. R. Sutton, R. Boland, M. Clark, S. Friedman, K. Brummel-Smith, and G. P. Eleazar. 2000. Hospitalization in the program of all-inclusive care for the elderly (PACE): Rates, concomitants, and predictors. *Journal of the American Geriatrics Society* 48(11):1373-1380.

Wilkerson, L., and D. M. Irby. 1998. Strategies for improving teaching practices: A comprehensive approach to faculty development. *Academic Medicine* 73(4):387-396.

Williams, R. S., H. F. Willard, and R. Snyderman. 2003. Personalized health planning. *Science* 300:549.

Wolf, D. A. 2001. Population change: Friend or foe of the chronic care system? *Health Affairs* 20(6):28-42.

Wolf, M. 2002. Clinical research career development: The individual perspective. *Academic Medicine* 77(11):1084-1088.

Wong, M. D., M. F. Shapiro, W. J. Boscardin, and S. L. Ettner. 2002. Contribution of major diseases to disparities in mortality. *New England Journal of Medicine* 347(20):1585-1592.

Writing Group for the Women's Health Initiative Investigators. 2002. Risks and benefits of estrogen plus progestin in healthy postmenopausal women: Principal results from the women's health initiative randomized controlled trial. *Journal of the American Medical Association* 288(3):321-333.

Yegian, J. 2003. Tiered Hospital Networks. *Health Affairs* Web Exclusive. Online. www.healthaffairs.org/WebExclusives/CHCF_Web_Excl_031903.htm.

Young, J. Q., and J. M. Coffman. 1998. Overview of graduate medical education: Funding streams, policy problems, and options for reform. *Western Journal of Medicine* 168(5):428-436.

Zelman, W. N., D. Blazer, J. M. Gower, P. O. Bumgarner, and L. M. Cancilla. 1999. Issues for academic health centers to consider before implementing a balanced-scorecard effort. *Academic Medicine* 74(12):1269-1277.

Zuckerman, S., G. Bazzoli, A. Davidoff, and A. LoSasso. 2001. How did safety-net hospitals cope in the 1990s? *Health Affairs* 20(4):159-168.

APPENDIX A

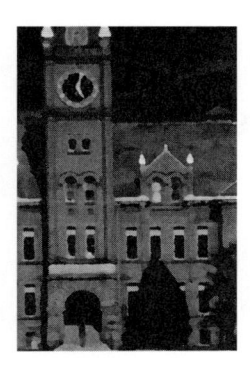

ACADEMIC HEALTH CENTERS: ALL THE SAME, ALL DIFFERENT, OR...

Report Prepared for
The Committee on the Roles of Academic Health Centers
in the 21st Century

Presented by:
Gerard Anderson, Ph.D.
The Johns Hopkins University Bloomberg School of Public Health
July 30, 2002

OBJECTIVES

This analysis examines the variation in roles across academic health centers (AHCs) for calendar year 2000. Roles examined are research, education, patient care, and care for the poor and uninsured. The rates of change in these roles between 1990 and 2000 are compared. The objectives of the analysis are to:

- Determine whether there are natural groupings of AHCs.
- Compare the activities among (1) AHC hospitals, (2) large teaching hospitals, and (3) small teaching hospitals.

DEFINITIONS

For purposes of this analysis, the following definitions are used:

Academic health center (AHC)
— Consists of a medical school and only one primary teaching hospital.
— The primary teaching hospital is determined based on data showing where most of the residents are trained. Data on other affiliated teaching hospitals are not included in the definition of an AHC. Some expert judgment was also involved in choosing the primary teaching hospital. A primary teaching hospital could not be established for osteopathic medical schools.
— Data from nursing, public health, and other related health professions schools, if they exist, are included in the definition of the AHC.

Hospital classification
— Large teaching hospital—not the primary affiliate of a medical school and has more than 0.25 residents per bed.
— Small teaching hospital—not the primary affiliate of a medical school, and has an Accreditation Council for Graduate Medical Education (ACGME) approved residency program and 0.25 or fewer residents per bed.
— Private hospital—includes both nonprofit and for-profit hospitals.
— Freestanding AHC—not a component of a larger university; primary activity is as an academic medical center.
— University-based AHC—combine the American Association of Medical Colleges (AAMC) definitions of related/proximate and related/distant institutions. Proximate medical schools are located

in the same city as the parent university; distant medical schools are not located in the same city as the parent university.

National Institutes of Health (NIH) funds—include direct and indirect payments.

Graduate Medical Education (GME) payments—include only direct graduate medical education payments from Medicare Cost Reports worksheet E3, Part IV.

Small metropolitan statistical area (MSA)—an area with fewer than 1 million inhabitants.

AHC top 50 ranking
— AHCs were ranked based on the level of:
  - Total NIH funding
  - Total Medicare disproportionate share (DSH) funding
  - Total direct Medicare GME funding
— AHCs were then classified based on whether they were in the top 50 in none, one, two, or all three above categories (for example, top 50 in both NIH and GME funding).

Dispersion—defined as the ratio of the value of the academic medical center at the 75th percentile to the value of the academic medical center at the 25th percentile.
— Low dispersion—ratio of the 75th percentile to the 25th percentile is less than 2.0.
— Medium dispersion—ratio of the 75th percentile to the 25th percentile is 2.0 to 2.9
— High dispersion—ratio of the 75th percentile to the 25th percentile is 3.0 or greater.

Margins

The Medicare Payment Advisory Commission (MedPAC) calculated three types of margins for this analysis that are included in Tables A-1 and A-2: Medicare hospital inpatient margins excluding direct GME payments and costs, overall Medicare margins including direct GME payments and costs, and total hospital margins. These calculations use 1999 data and are based on a slightly different sample of hospitals.

The margins are calculated as revenues minus costs divided by revenues. The Medicare margins are based on Medicare-allowed costs. The overall Medicare margin includes the largest Medicare services: acute inpatient, outpatient, rehabilitation, and psychiatric units; skilled nursing facility; and home health agency. It also reflects Medicare payments for direct GME and bad debts. The total margin reflects the relationship of all hospital revenues to all costs (including Medicare-nonallowed costs).

METHODS

Roles

As noted, this analysis examines four activities of academic health centers, which are measured using available indicators: research, education, patient care, and indigent care. Analysis of the data is presented by role. Only statistically significant results are discussed. Statistically significant results that are obvious, such as hospitals with more beds also having a higher average daily census, are not discussed.

Data Sources

The following data sources are used in this analysis:

- Medicare Hospital Cost Reports for FY 1990 and 1999
- American Hospital Association Annual Surveys for 1990 and 2000
- NIH data on trends in awards to medical schools 1990 and 2000
- American Association of Health Service Library Surveys, 1990 and 2000
- American Association of Colleges of Nursing Annual Survey, 1994 and 2001, special runs performed for this project
- AAMC, special runs performed for this project.
- MedPAC, special runs performed for this project

DATA ANALYSIS

These analyses are based on 120 AHC hospitals and 119 medical schools. Cost data for FY 1990 and 1999 are based on 117 hospitals.

- Statistics provided for all variables as of the calendar year 2000:
  — Mean
  — 25th percentile
  — Median
  — 75th percentile
  — Total rate of change between 1990 and 2000

- Characteristics of Academic health center hospitals:
  — Size
    - Fewer than 500 beds
    - Greater than or equal to 500 beds
  — Ownership
    - Government
    - Private (nonprofit or for-profit)

- MSA
  - Fewer than 1 million inhabitants
  - More than 1 million inhabitants
- Location
  - Northeast
  - South
  - Midwest
  - West

• Characteristics of Medical Schools
  - Date founded
    - Before 1960
    - During or after 1960
  - Type
    - Free standing
    - University based

• Top 50 ranking by funding category
  - NIH, GME, and DSH
  - NIH and GME only
  - NIH and DSH only
  - GME and DSH only
  - NIH only
  - GME only
  - DSH only
  - Not top 50 in any category

• Differences among groups calculated using analysis of variance (ANOVA). Statistically significant differences ($p < .05$) are shown in bold in the tables.

RESULTS

The empirical results are reported as follows:

- Table A-1—Dispersion Across the AHCs by Activity, 2000
- Table A-2—Comparison of the AHCs by Characteristic, 2000
- Table A-3—Comparison by Top 50 in Funding Criteria, 2000
- Table A-4—Rate of Change in Activity by Statistical Dispersion Category, 1990–2000
- Table A-5—Rate of Change in Activity by AHC Characteristic, 1990–2000

- Table A-6—Rate of Change in Activity by Top 50 Funding Criteria, 1990–2000
- Table A-7—Comparison of Hospitals by Teaching Program Size, 2000
- Table A-8—Rate of Change in Activity by Teaching Program Size, 1990–2000
- Table A-9—Provision of Specialized Services by Teaching Status
- Table A-10—Comparison of Market Share by Teaching Program Size

SUMMARY OF RESULTS BY ROLE

Research

- The greatest disparity among AHCs occurs in level of research funding.
- Certain categories of AHCs received more research funding than others.
- NIH funding increased 126 percent at the mean AHC between 1990 and 2000.
- While there were differences in the rate of increase in research funding across AHCs between 1990 and 2000, there were few statistically significant differences by type of AHC.

Education

- In general, educational variables showed moderate to low dispersion and generally did not vary systematically by type of AHC.
- The number of residents increased by 35 percent and the number of nursing students increased by 9 percent between 1990 and 2000.
- GME payments per resident actually declined from 1990 to 2000 by 3 percent.
- There was little systematic change between 1990 and 2000 in the level of commitment to education by category of AHC.

Patient Care

- Patient care services showing moderate dispersion across AHCs were total emergency room visits, total outpatient visits, Medicare inpatient days, Medicaid inpatient days, and percent Medicaid inpatient days. All the other patient care services had low dispersion. The committee noted the low dispersion in percent Medicare days.
- Among AHCs, the greatest dispersion among patient care services was seen between AHCs with large and small hospitals and between hospitals located in the Northeast and those located elsewhere.

- Between 1990 and 2000, the most rapid increase occurred in outpatient and emergency room visits.
- On most patient care variables, there were no systematic differences in the rate of change between 1990 and 2000 by category of AHC.

Disproportionate Share
- There was high dispersion in DSH payments per Medicare discharge.
- Higher DSH payments per Medicare discharge were received by AHCs located in larger MSAs and by public AHCs.
- Mean DSH payments per Medicare discharge increased 91 percent between 1990 and 2000. There were no systematic differences by category of AHC.

Market Share
- Hospitals were classified into four groups—AHC hospitals, large teaching, small teaching, and nonteaching hospitals. AHC hospitals generally provide more education, patient care, and DSH share than the other types of hospitals.
- AHC hospitals generally provide more education, patient care, and disproportionate share than the other types of hospitals.
- The level of commitment to education did not change among AHC hospitals, large teaching hospitals, and small teaching hospitals between 1990 and 2000.
- While AHCs are only 3 percent of all hospitals, they provide a much larger proportion of training and patient care. However, they are not the majority (> 50 percent) producer of any services. They provide 48 percent of residency training.
- The market share of AHCs increased between 1990 and 2000.

Notes on Table A-1

Dispersion Across the AHCs by Activity

Research
- The greatest dispersion across the AHCs for all variables occurs with respect to the level of NIH funding. In 2000, the AHC at the 25th percentile received $11.6 million in NIH funding, compared with $90.7 million for the AHC at the 75th percentile. In other words, the AHC at the 75th percentile received 7.8 times more NIH funding than the AHC at the 25th percentile. Using this measure of dispersion, this is the indicator with the largest variation of all variables analyzed.
- Among all indicators studied, the second-greatest amount of dispersion occurs with respect to NIH funding per full-time equivalent (FTE)

faculty member. At the 25th percentile, the average faculty member receives $27,244 in NIH funding, compared with $86,769 at the 75th percentile.

Education

- Across AHCs, there is moderate dispersion in the total number of residents and total clinical faculty.
- Across academic health centers, there is relatively low variance in biological Medical College Admissions Test (MCAT) scores, percentage family practice residents, percentage internal medicine residents, percentage pediatrics residents, percentage primary care residents, number of residents per bed, GME payments per resident, number of nursing school graduates, and library recurring expenditures.

Patient Care Services

- None of the patient care services showed high dispersion across the AHC hospitals.

  - Moderate dispersion was demonstrated in:
    — Total emergency room visits
    — Total outpatient visits
    — Total Medicare inpatient days
    — Total Medicaid inpatient days
    — Percent Medicaid inpatient days
  - Low dispersion was demonstrated in
    — Average daily census
    — Total hospital inpatient beds
    — Occupancy rate
    — Total inpatient days
    — Percent Medicare inpatient days
    — Medicare case mix index
    — Total FTE personnel
    — FTE nurses per 1,000 inpatient days
    — Total FTE personnel per 1,000 inpatient days
    — Length of stay (overall, Medicare, Medicaid)

- There was high dispersion in disproportionate share payments per Medicare discharge.

Notes on Table A-2

Comparison of the AHC by Characteristic

AHC Characteristics

- AHCs in larger MSAs, AHC hospitals with more than 500 beds, and

AHCs with medical schools founded before 1960 all received more total NIH funding than their counterparts in 2000.

Research
- There was no difference in the level of total NIH funding between freestanding and university-based AHCs or between public and private institutions.
- NIH funding per FTE faculty member was greater in larger MSAs, AHCs with larger hospitals, medical schools founded prior to 1960, and AHCs located in the West.
- No difference in the level of NIH funding per FTE faculty member was detected between public and private institutions or between freestanding and university-based AHCs.

Education
- AHCs in large MSAs and medical schools founded prior to 1960 had higher resident-to-bed ratios and more recurring library expenditures.
- AHCs located in the West had the highest ratios of residents to beds.
- AHCs located in the Northeast received the highest level of GME funding per resident.

Patient Care
- AHC hospitals located in small MSAs had a higher percentage of Medicare patients and lower Medicare overall and inpatient margins.
- Public AHC hospitals had a smaller percentage of Medicare patients and a larger percentage of Medicaid patients than private hospitals.
- Smaller AHC hospitals had more FTEs per 1,000 inpatient days, shorter overall and Medicare lengths of stay, and a lower Medicare case mix.
- AHC hospitals whose medical school was founded before 1960 had more nurses per 1,000 inpatient days.
- AHC hospitals located in the Northeast had the longest lengths of stay (overall, and Medicare), fewest FTE nurses per 1,000 inpatient day, fewest FTE personnel per 1,000 inpatient days, lowest percent of Medicaid days, highest occupancy rate, and highest Medicare overall and Medicare inpatient margins.

DSH Funds
- AHC hospitals located in larger MSAs received higher DSH payments per Medicare discharge.
- Public AHC hospitals received higher DSH payments per Medicare beneficiary.
- AHC hospitals located in the West received more DSH payments per Medicare discharge.

Notes on Table A-3

Comparison by Top 50 in Funding Criteria

- AHCs with the highest resident-to-bed ratios were in the top 50 in GME only while AHCs that were in the top 50 in DSH only had the lowest ratios.
- AHCs that are in the top 50 on GME only received the highest GME payments per resident while AHCs in the top 50 in NIH only received the lowest.
- AHCs that are in the top 50 in both NIH and GME had the most nursing graduates, while those that were not in the top 50 on any category had the least.
- AHC hospitals that were in the top 50 for DSH only had the highest percentage of Medicaid days, while those that are in the top 50 in NIH and GME had the lowest.
- AHC hospitals with the highest occupancy rates were in the top 50 for GME only, while hospitals with the lowest occupancy rates were not in the top 50 in any category.

Notes on Table A-4

Rate of Change in Activity by Statistical Dispersion Category (1990-2000)

Research

- The mean increase in NIH funding for all AHCs between 1990 and 2000 was 126 percent. The increase in the level of funding varied considerably. The AHC at the 25th percentile had an NIH funding increase of 60 percent while the AHC at the 75th percentile had an NIH funding increase of 161 percent.

Education

- At AHC hospitals, the total number of residents increased an average of 33 percent between 1990 and 2000. The number of residents increased 1 percent in the AHC hospital at the 25th percentile and 44 percent in the AHC hospital at the 75th percentile
- The resident-per-bed ratio increased by 35 percent between 1990 and 2000. The ratio in the AHC hospital at the 25th percentile increased 12 percent while that in the AHC hospital of the 75th percentile increased 50 percent.
- The mean of the distribution of percentage changes across all institutions that graduated nurses in both 1990 and 2000 was 9 percent. At the

25th percentile, the decline was 17 percent, while at the 75th percentile the increase was 12 percent.

Patient Care

- Between 1990 and 2000, the greatest increase occurred in outpatient visits, followed by emergency room visits and total FTE personnel per 1,000 inpatient days.

Patient Care—DSH

- The mean AHC hospital received 91 percent more in DSH payments per Medicare discharge in 2000 than in 1990. The 25th percentile AHC hospital received 31 percent more, while the 75th percentile AHC hospital received 123 percent more.

Notes on Table A-5

Rate of Change in Activity by AHC Characteristic (1990-2000)

- On most educational variables, the rate of increase between 1990 and 2000 did not vary systematically by category of AHC. The one exception was total residents, which increased more rapidly at private hospitals.
- There were few statistically significant differences in the rate of increase from 1990 to 2000 by category of AHC hospital for patient care variables. The one major exception was private hospitals, which had greater increases in the number of outpatient visits and total FTE personnel and showed a more rapid decline in overall length of stay. It is also noted that private hospitals had a statistically significant increase in hospital beds as compared with public hospitals, which experienced a decline in that time period.
- AHC hospitals in the Midwest showed the greatest decline in overall length of stay (LOS) while those in the Northeast showed the greatest overall decline in Medicare LOS.
- AHCs whose medical schools were founded before 1960 saw their NIH funds increase more rapidly than AHCs whose medical schools were founded during or after 1960.
- There were no statistically significant differences in rate of increase in NIH funding by:
  — Level of funding in 1990
  — MSA size
  — Number of hospital beds
  — University based vs. freestanding
  — Ownership (public vs. private)
  — Region

Notes on Table A-6

Rate of Change in Activity by Top 50 Funding Criteria

- AHC hospitals in the top 50 in NIH and GME funding showed the greatest decline in percent Medicaid inpatient days.
- There were no statistically significant differences in rates of increase in any of the other research, patient care, or education variables by funding category.

Notes on Table A-7

Comparison of Hospitals by Teaching Program Size

Research
No data available.

Education
Compared with the other teaching hospitals, AHC hospitals had:
- More total residents
- Higher-resident-to bed ratios
- Lower Medicare GME payments per resident

Patient Care
Compared with other teaching hospitals, AHC hospitals were much larger. They had:

- Higher daily censuses
- More emergency room visits
- More outpatient visits
- More hospital beds
- Higher occupancy rates
- More Medicare days
- More Medicaid days
- More total inpatient days
- Higher proportion of Medicaid days
- Higher Medicare case mix
- Longer overall, Medicare, and Medicaid lengths of stay
- Lower percentage of Medicare days.

- Given their higher intensity of care, it is somewhat surprising that there were no statistically significant differences in number of FTE nurses per 1,000 inpatient days.

Patient Care—DSH Funds

Compared with other teaching hospitals, AHC hospitals received higher DSH payments

Notes on Table A-8

Rate of Change in Activity by Teaching Program Size (1990-2000)

- The only statistically significant difference in the rate of change between 1990 and 2000 on any of the education variables among the three groups was in residents per bed. AHCs had the smallest rate of change among the three groups of teaching hospitals.
- Between 1990 and 2000, AHC hospitals had:
  — Smallest reduction in hospital beds
  — Smallest reduction in average daily census
  — Smallest reduction in percent of Medicare inpatient days
  — Greatest overall decline in percent of Medicaid days
  — Largest increase in Medicare case mix index
  — Smallest reduction in overall length of stay
- There were no statistically significant differences in the rate of change between 1990 and 2000 in DSH payments.

Notes on Table A-9

Provision of Specialized Services by Teaching Status

- AHC hospitals represented 3 percent of all hospitals in 2000.
- In no category did they provide a majority of services. However, they:
  — Trained 48 percent of all residents
  — Provided 20 percent of Medicaid inpatient days
  — Provided 16 percent of Medicaid hospital discharges
  — Provided 13 percent of all inpatient days
  — Provided 11 percent of all hospital discharges
  — Represented 10 percent of all hospital beds
  — Provided 9 percent of all Medicare days
  — Provided 8 percent of all Medicare discharges
- The percent of specialty services available at AHC hospitals shown in the table measures the availability of services, not the use of services. The services for which more than 20 percent are available at AHC hospitals are burn unit, transplant services, pediatric unit, and positron emission tomography (PET) scanner.

Notes on Table A-10

Comparison of Market Share by Teaching Program Size

- In 1990, AHCs represented 2 percent of hospitals, 7 percent of hospital beds, and 8 percent of total discharges. By 1999, AHCs represented 3 percent of all hospitals, 10 percent of all hospital beds, and 11 percent of total discharges. The AHC share of Medicare and Medicaid discharges increased similarly.

In general, AHCs and major teaching hospitals increased their market share between 1990 and 1999, while small teaching and nonteaching hospitals lost market share.

APPENDIX A TABLES

TABLE A-1 Dispersion Across the AHCs by Activity, 2000

All Academic Health Centers, 2000

Variable	Mean	25th Percentile	Median	75th Percentile	Ratio 75th Percentile/ 25th Percentile
NIH Funding	$62,689,524	$11,649,000	$42,219,000	$90,728,000	7.8
Full-Time Clinical Science Faculty	717	364	564	919	2.5
NIH Funding per full-time basic science and clinical faculty	$63,403	$27,244	$56,223	$86,769	3.2
Biological Science MCAT	$10	$10	$10	$11	1.1
Total Residents—Hospital	308	198	278	410	2.1
% Family Practice Residents	7	5	5	7	1.4
% Internal Medicine Residents	23	17	20	22	1.3
% Pediatric Residents	9	7	9	10	1.3
% Primary Care Residents	39	29	35	38	1.3
Residents per Bed	0.59	0.44	0.59	0.74	1.7
GME $ per Resident	$65,200	$47,077	$59,794	$76,713	1.6
Nursing Graduates	169	115	159	219	1.9
Library Recurring Expenses	$2,861,640	$1,986,795	$2,714,715	$3,581,601	1.8

Average Daily Census	428	275	396	516	1.9
Total ER Visits	57,690	34,332	50,979	67,586	2.0
Total Outpatient Visits	419,145	236,563	374,944	544,123	2.3
Total Hospital Beds	532	370	489	656	1.8
Occupancy Rate	69%	64%	69%	77%	1.2
Medicare Inpatient Days—Total Hospital	40,331	22,634	35,576	51,509	2.3
Medicaid IP Days—Total Hospital	27,970	11,934	21,898	34,516	2.9
Total IP Days—Hospital	135,726	84,546	130,290	163,025	1.9
% MCR IP Days (Hospital)	30%	23%	30%	37%	1.6
% MCD IP Days (Hospital)	20%	13%	19%	26%	2.0
Medicare Case Mix Index	1.77	1.63	1.78	1.88	1.2
FTE Total Personnel	3,774	2,561	3,266	4,619	1.8
FTE Nurses per 1,000 IP Days	6.8	5.6	6.7	7.5	1.3
Total FTE per 1,000 IP Days	25.4	24.3	25.4	29.3	1.2
Overall Length of Stay (LOS)	5.8	5.2	5.7	6.2	1.2
Medicare LOS	6.5	5.9	6.3	7.1	1.2
Medicaid LOS	6.3	5.0	5.9	7.0	1.4
Medicare Inpatient (Margin)*	20.6	14.6	19.0	26.1	1.8
Overall Medicare (Margin)**	11.3	5.1	10.6	16.5	3.3
Total Hospital (Margin)	3.2	-2.3	1.3	4.5	-2.0
DSH Payment per Medicare dischg.	$1,454	$697	$1,324	$2,066	3.0

* Excludes direct GME payments and costs.
** Includes direct GME payments and costs.

TABLE A-2-1 Comparison of the AHCs by Characteristic, 2000

All Academic Medical Centers, 2000
(bold values differ by p <.05)

Variable	All	< 1 mil.	≥ 1 mil.
NIH Funding	$62,689,524	**$40,435,000**	**$77,216,782**
Full-Time Clinical Science Faculty	717	**478**	**879**
NIH Funding per full-time basic science and clinical faculty	$63,403	**$52,644**	**$70,525**
Biological Science MCAT	10.2	9.9	10.5
Total Residents—Hospital	483	361	564
% of Family Practice Residents	7	9	6
% Internal Medicine Residents	23	20	24
% Pediatric Residents	9	9	10
% Primary Care Residents	39	38	40
Residents per Bed	0.59	**0.51**	**0.64**
GME $ per resident	$65,200	$63,248	$66,510
Total Clinical Faculty	674	473	807
Nursing Graduates	169	160	177
Library Recurring Expense	$2,861,640	**$2,472,726**	**$3,146,843**
Average daily census	428	**367**	**469**
Total ER visits	57,690	52,591	61,090
Total outpatient visits	419,145	399,889	431,982
Total Hospital Beds	532	**482**	**566**
Occupancy Rate	69%	69%	69%
Medicare IP Days—Total Hospital	40,331	40,678	40,098
Medicaid IP Days—Total Hospital	27,970	23,597	30,906
Total IP Days—Hospital	135,726	121,570	145,231
% MCR IP Days (Hospital)	30%	**34%**	**27%**
% MCD IP Days (Hospital)	20%	19%	22%
Medicare Casemix Index	1.77	1.78	1.76
FTE total personnel	3,774	**3,195**	**4,160**
FTE Nurses per 1,000 IP Days	6.8	6.9	6.7
Total FTE per 1,000 IP Days	25.4	24.5	25.9
Overall Length of Stay (LOS)	5.8	5.7	5.9
Medicare LOS	6.5	6.3	6.7
Medicaid LOS	6.3	6.0	6.6
Medicare Inpatient (Margins)	20.6	**17.2**	**22.7**
Overall Medicare (Margins)	11.3	**9.6**	**12.3**
Total Hospital (Margins)	3.2	4.9	2.2
Medicare Inpatient (% Margins at Loss)	2	4	0
Overall Medicare (% Margins at Loss)	15	13	16
Total Hospital (% Margins at Loss)	36	29	42
DSH Payment per Medicare dischg.	$1,454	**$1,156**	**$1,655**

APPENDIX A

	1 AMC in MSA	2+ AMCs in MSA	Private	Public	<500 beds	500+ beds
	$54,008,947	$77,485,961	$68,806,056	$51,475,881	**$35,676,712**	**$88,373,836**
	592	**939**	**786**	**586**	**497**	**920**
	$62,315	$65,301	$61,757	$66,494	$50,404	$75,549
	10	10.4	10.1	10.4		
	267	**382**	447	745	386	570
	8	7	9	6		
	21	23	21	23		
	9	10	10	9		
	38	40	40	38		
	0.54	**0.66**	0.56	0.64	0.61	0.56
	$60,123	**$74,265**	$65,889	$63,921	$63,768	$66,759
	692	745	560	776		
	167	172	164	176	159	177
	$2,743,769	$3,075,081	$2,796,980	$2,969,405	**$2,399,390**	**$3,257,853**
	402	473	446	396	**270**	**576**
	55,955	60,688	54,976	62,732	**45,191**	**69,383**
	414,047	427,950	405,256	444,937	**331,629**	**501,014**
	505	580	**565**	**472**	358	722
	68%	71%	69%	69%	68%	70%
	37,602	45,204	**47,811**	**26,466**	27,869	53,905
	25,214	32,890	25,527	32,498	**17,387**	**39,497**
	125,565	153,870	143,713	120,920	**89,783**	**185,771**
	31%	29%	**33%**	**24%**	31%	29%
	19%	22%	**17%**	**26%**	20%	21%
	1.79	1.73	1.79	1.72	**1.73**	**1.81**
	3,489	4,265	3,983	3,386	**2,610**	**4,862**
	7.0	6.5	6.6	7.2	7.0	6.6
	25.0	26.1	24.9	26.2	**26.8**	**24.1**
	5.8	5.8	5.7	6.0	**5.6**	**6.0**
	6.4	6.8	6.5	6.6	**6.3**	**6.8**
	6.1	6.8	6.5	6.1	5.9	6.9
	19.8	22.9	20.1	20.8		
	11.4	10.8	11.3	11.3		
	3.6	2.2	1.5	4		
	3	0	2	2		
	11	24	13	16		
	33	42	43	30		
	$1,348	$1,645	**$1,188**	**$1,948**	$1,408	$1,505

TABLE A-2-2 Comparison of the AHCs by Characteristic, 2000

All Academic Medical Centers, 2000
(bold values differ by p <.05)

	Post-1960	Pre-1960
NIH Funding	**$24,807,009**	**$79,311,940**
Full-Time Clinical Science Faculty	**417**	**847**
NIH Funding per full-time basic science and clinical faculty	**$43,955**	**$71,604**
Biological Science MCAT	9.9	10.4
Total Residents—Hospital	375	529
% of Family Practice Residents	9	7
% Internal Medicine Residents	24	22
% Pediatric Residents	9	10
% Primary Care Residents	42	39
Residents per Bed	**0.48**	**0.63**
GME $ per resident	$62,776	$65,687
Total Clinical Faculty	421	782
Nursing Graduates	154	175
Library Recurring Expense	**$2,413,861**	**$3,034,781**
Average daily census	**366**	**457**
Total ER visits	60,333	56,368
Total outpatient visits	371,179	442,435
Total Hospital Beds	**472**	**562**
Occupancy Rate	68%	70%
Medicare IP Days—Total Hospital	38,108	41,705
Medicaid IP Days—Total Hospital	**21,364**	**30,531**
Total IP Days—Hospital	**117,013**	**144,461**
% MCR IP Days (Hospital)	32%	29%
% MCD IP Days (Hospital)	18%	21%
Medicare Casemix Index	1.75	1.78
FTE total personnel	**3,189**	**4,039**
FTE Nurses per 1,000 IP Days	**6.4**	**7.0**
Total FTE per 1,000 IP Days	24.5	25.7
Overall Length of Stay (LOS)	5.6	5.9
Medicare LOS	6.3	6.6
Medicaid LOS	5.8	6.6
Medicare Inpatient (Margins)	20.8	20.2
Overall Medicare (Margins)	10.8	12.9
Total Hospital (Margins)	3.9	1
Medicare Inpatient (% Margins at Loss)	0	6
Overall Medicare (% Margins at Loss)	15	11
Total Hospital (% Margins at Loss)	43	30
DSH Payment per Medicare dischg.	$1,323	$1,471

APPENDIX A

	Freestanding	University-Based	Northeast	South	Midwest	West
	$48,119,458	$66,981,588	$72,009,621	$53,113,674	$52,777,910	$88,502,882
	621	743	**1,002**	**579**	**599**	**799**
	$55,531	$65,413	**$62,720**	**$56,978**	**$56,521**	**$94,812**
	10.1	10.3	10.5	10	10.1	10.6
	514	474	604	416	441	528
	8	7	4	8	8	9
	22	23	27	19	21	24
	9	9	9	10	10	10
	39	39	40	37	39	43
	0.58	0.58	**0.66**	**0.53**	**0.54**	**0.70**
	$60,017	$66,059	**$76,985**	**$63,534**	**$62,679**	**$55,195**
	611	690	797	657	580	678
	168	169	150	172	179	168
	$2,910,297	$2,848,585	$3,014,322	$2,844,958	$2,501,413	$3,262,530
	422	432	**556**	**407**	**380**	**353**
	52,715	58,859	61,182	59,008	48,455	65,242
	392,005	428,558	474,213	362,008	399,546	505,465
	527	537	578	560	498	456
	67%	69%	**76%**	**66%**	**67%**	**69%**
	35,911	41,848	**53,355**	**37,868**	**42,882**	**21,080**
	26,270	28,155	28,135	33,420	19,840	29,066
	128,791	138,107	162,502	136,095	122,904	115,667
	28%	31%	**33%**	**28%**	**35%**	**19%**
	22%	19%	**16%**	**24%**	**17%**	**24%**
	1.78	1.77	1.84	1.77	1.74	1.70
	3,467	3,865	4,445	3,476	3,622	3,658
	6.6	6.9	**5.9**	**6.8**	**7.1**	**7.9**
	24.3	25.6	**23.4**	**24.2**	**26.6**	**29.5**
	6.2	5.7	**6.5**	**5.9**	**5.4**	**5.3**
	6.8	6.4	**7.3**	**6.5**	**6.2**	**5.9**
	6.7	6.3	**6.4**	7.0	5.6	5.9
	20.8	19.7	**25.4**	**19.1**	**15.9**	**21.4**
	12	**15.3**	**15.3**	**10.4**	**6.3**	**11.3**
	0.9	**2.1**	**0.9**	**2.1**	**7.2**	**2.9**
	2	0	0	3	0	7
	11	24	4	12	26	27
	33	**52**	29	43	34	20
	$1,741	$1,344	**$1,338**	**$1,670**	**$954**	**$2,019**

TABLE A-3 Comparison by Top 50 in Funding Criteria, 2000

All Academic Health Centers, 2000
(bold values differ by p <.05)

Variable	Top 50, NIH, GME, DSH	Top 50, NIH and GME	Top 50, NIH and DSH
NIH Funding	**$132,518,250**	**$120,947,333**	**$112,967,333**
Full-Time Clinical Science Faculty	**1,130**	**1,416**	**841**
NIH Funding per full-time basic science and clinical faculty	**$99,137**	**$85,417**	**$118,950**
Biological MCAT	11	10.6	10.6
Total Residents—Hospital	773	564	515
% of Family Practice Residents	5	5	5
% Internal Medicine Residents	24	22	16
% Pediatrics Residents	10	7	11
% Primary Care Residents	39	34	32
Residents per Bed	**0.68**	**0.73**	**0.55**
GME $ per resident	**$69,338**	**$80,838**	**$50,576**
Total Clinical Faculty	1058	954	767
Nursing Graduates	**175**	**223**	**189**
Library Recurring Expense	**$3,635,405**	**$3,550,124**	**$3,094,337**
Average daily census	**678**	**562**	**462**
Total ER visits	**80,126**	**71,880**	**54,633**
Total outpatient visits	**624,288**	**626,292**	**451,506**
Total Hospital Beds	**829**	**639**	**584**
Occupancy Rate	**74%**	**76%**	**71%**
Medicare IP Days—Total Hospital	**66,570**	**47,243**	**47,246**
Medicaid IP Days—Total Hospital	**54,998**	**23,570**	**26,408**
Total IP Days—Hospital	**223,239**	**176,139**	**150,935**
% MCR IP Days (Hospital)	30%	28%	30%
% MCD IP Days (Hospital)	**25%**	**13%**	**19%**
Medicare Casemix Index	1.76	1.81	1.88
FTE total personnel	**6,286**	**5,355**	**3,736**
FTE Nurses per 1,000 IP Days	7.3	7.4	6.1
Total FTE per 1,000 IP Days	27.0	27.2	22.8
Overall Length of Stay (LOS)	6.0	5.6	5.8
Medicare LOS	6.8	6.7	6.4
Medicaid LOS	7.6	5.5	6.6
DSH Payment per Medicare dischg.	$1,535	$1,369	$1,361

	Top 50, GME and DSH	Top 50, NIH	Top 50, GME	Top 50, DSH	None
	$23,770,455	$113,201,583	$25,971,667	$17,040,333	$17,734,657
	590	926	453	356	382
	$39,171	$103,314	$53,477	$32,731	$36,754
	10.1	10.6	10.1	9.7	9.8
	351	591	386	322	353
	6	10	4	11	9
	23	22	19	21	23
	9	10	8	9	10
	38	31	41	42	
	0.59	0.70	0.75	0.43	0.48
	$81,584	$47,154	$91,343	$58,327	$58,790
	905	832	445	362	378
	178	190	185	162	129
	$3,159,827	$3,718,533	$2,442,508	$2,249,832	$1,933,196
	423	369	305	381	293
	60,910	46,276	42,728	57,950	48,715
	385,021	443,800	316,424	339,509	298,022
	574	429	369	542	372
	69%	66%	77%	68%	64%
	47,647	27,931	26,354	36,490	27,946
	32,032	15,004	20,865	41,660	14,639
	144,267	101,960	103,805	131,504	87,575
	33%	28%	26%	29%	32%
	23%	15%	22%	31%	18%
	1.68	1.83	1.70	1.76	1.74
	3,919	3,576	2,767	2,985	2,458
	6.7	7.5	6.9	6.6	6.5
	26.2	27.7	25.6	22.2	25.2
	5.9	5.7	5.7	5.7	5.8
	6.7	6.0	6.8	6.3	6.5
	6.2	6.6	5.1	6.8	5.9
	$1,697	$1,141	$1,843	$1,938	$1,257

TABLE A-4 Rate of Change in Activity by Statistical Dispersion Category, 1990-2000

All Academic Health Centers
Percent Change 1990-2000

Variable	Mean	25th Percentile	Median	75th Percentile
% Chg. - NIH Funding	126%	60%	107%	161%
% Chg. - Total Residents—Hospital	33%	1%	22%	44%
% Chg. - Residents per Bed	35%	12%	26%	50%
% Chg. - GME $ per resident	−3%	−24%	−8%	9%
% Chg. - Linrary Recurring Expense	81%	48%	71%	98%
% Chg. - Nursing Graduates*	9%	−17%	−9%	12%
% Chg. - Average daily census	−2%	−25%	−10%	10%
% Chg. - Total ER visits	54%	3%	30%	74%
% Chg. - Total outpatient visits	133%	19%	81%	172%
% Chg. - Total Hospital Beds	0%	−15%	−3%	10%
% Chg. - Occupancy Rate	−8%	−12%	−7%	−1%
% Chg. - Medicare IP Days—Total Hospital	−7%	−28%	−13%	3%
% Chg. - Medicaid IP Days—Total Hospital	−10%	−39%	−19%	3%
% Chg. - Total IP Days—Hospital	−10%	−25%	−13%	1%
% Chg. - % MCR IP Days (Hospital)	0%	−3%	0%	3%
% Chg. - % MCD IP Days (Hospital)	−2%	−6%	−1%	3%
% Chg. - Medicare Casemix Index	20%	12%	20%	29%
% Chg. - FTE total personnel	26%	4%	22%	39%
% Chg. - FTE Nurses per 1,000 IP Days	33%	11%	29%	51%
% Chg. - Total FTE per 1,000 IP Days	35%	13%	33%	50%
% Chg. - Overall Length of Stay (LOS)	−17%	−27%	−20%	−9%
% Chg. - Medicare LOS	−31%	−37%	−32%	−26%
% Chg. - Medicaid LOS	−4%	−27%	−13%	10%
% Chg. - DSH Payment per Medicare dischg.	91%	31%	65%	123%

* Calculated by dividing the sum of all percentage changes by the number of institutions (98) with nursing graduate data in both 1990 and 2000.

TABLE A-5 IS ON THE NEXT PAGE

TABLE A-5-1 Rate of Change in Activity by AHC Characteristic, 1990-2000

All Academic Health Centers
Percent Change 1990-2000
(bold values differ by p <.05)

	All (Mean)	< 1 mil.	≥ 1 mil.
% Chg. - NIH Funding	126%	142%	116%
% Chg. - Total Residents—Hospital	33%	39%	33%
% Chg. - Residents per Bed	35%	36%	35%
% Chg. - GME $ per resident	–3%	4%	–9%
% Chg. - Library Recurring Expense	81%	88%	75%
% Chg. - Nursing Graduates	9%	–2%	19%
% Chg. - Average daily census	–2%	5%	–7%
% Chg. - Total ER visits	54%	59%	51%
% Chg. - Total outpatient visits	133%	132%	133%
% Chg. - Total Hospital Beds	0%	3%	0%
% Chg. - Occupancy Rate	–8%	–7%	–9%
% Chg. - Medicare IP Days—Total Hospital	–7%	**3%**	**–11%**
% Chg. - Medicaid IP Days—Total Hospital	–10%	–3%	–12%
% Chg. - Total IP Days—Hospital	–10%	–5%	–12%
% Chg. - % MCR IP Days (Hospital)	0%	**1%**	**–1%**
% Chg. - % MCD IP Days (Hospital)	–2%	–1%	–3%
% Chg. - Casemix Index	20%	20%	20%
% Chg. - FTE total personnel	26%	31%	23%
% Chg. - FTE Nurses per 1000 IP Days	33%	30%	35%
% Chg. - Total FTE per 1000 IP Days	35%	31%	37%
% Chg. - Overall LOS	–17%	–16%	–17%
% Chg. - Medicare LOS	–31%	–32%	–30%
% Chg. - Medicaid LOS	–4%	0%	–6%
% Chg. - Disp Shr Payment per MCR dischg.	91%	87%	92%

APPENDIX A

1 AHC in MSA	2+ AHCs in MSA	Private	Public	<500 beds	500+ beds
137%	108%	126%	127%	131%	122%
35%	28%	**43%**	**20%**	34%	37%
34%	37%	39%	29%	43%	28%
−1%	−6%	−7%	2%	−1%	−7%
81%	80%	66%	93%	66%	94%
6%	17%	3%	20%	15%	4%
2%	**−10%**	0%	−6%	−7%	2%
49%	63%	66%	33%	38%	69%
135%	128%	**171%**	**61%**	107%	157%
2%	−4%	**5%**	**−6%**	**−4%**	**8%**
−9%	−7%	−9%	−7%	−7%	−9%
−7%	−6%	−8%	−2%	−6%	−5%
−10%	−12%	−2%	−22%	−14%	−3%
−9%	−13%	−6%	−14%	−13%	−4%
0%	−1%	**−1%**	**1%**	0%	−1%
−3%	−2%	−2%	−3%	−3%	−2%
22%	18%	19%	23%	20%	20%
30%	21%	**31%**	**18%**	24%	29%
33%	33%	33%	34%	32%	34%
32%	39%	36%	32%	38%	32%
−16%	−18%	**−20%**	**−11%**	−17%	−16%
−32%	−30%	−32%	−29%	−32%	−30%
−5%	−2%	−5%	−1%	−6%	−1%
85%	102%	95%	82%	83%	98%

TABLE A-5-2 Rate of Change in Activity by AHC Characteristic, 1990-2000

All Academic Health Centers
Percent Change 1990-2000
(bold values differ by p <.05)

	Post-1960	Pre-1960	Freestanding
% Chg. - NIH Funding	97%	139%	127%
% Chg. - Total Residents—Hospital	40%	30%	21%
% Chg. - Residents per Bed	40%	33%	26%
% Chg. - GME $ per resident	1%	−4%	−10%
% Chg. - Library Recurring Expense	94%	72%	84%
% Chg. - Nursing Graduates	−2%	14%	46%
% Chg. - Average daily census	4%	−5%	−3%
% Chg. - Total ER visits	52%	55%	59%
% Chg. - Total outpatient visits	125%	138%	142%
% Chg. - Total Hospital Beds	1%	0%	−1%
% Chg. - Occupancy Rate	−8%	−8%	−9%
% Chg. - Medicare IP Days—Total Hospital	−8%	−9%	−13%
% Chg. - Medicaid IP Days—Total Hospital	−20%	−6%	−9%
% Chg. - Total IP Days—Hospital	−8%	−11%	−13%
% Chg. - % MCR IP Days (Hospital)	0%	0%	−1%
% Chg. - % MCD IP Days (Hospital)	−4%	−2%	1%
% Chg. - Casemix Index	21%	20%	24%
% Chg. - FTE total personnel	31%	24%	20%
% Chg. - FTE Nurses per 1000 IP Days	26%	35%	25%
% Chg. - Total FTE per 1000 IP Days	33%	36%	28%
% Chg. - Overall LOS	−15%	−18%	−13%
% Chg. - Medicare LOS	−31%	−31%	−31%
% Chg. - Medicaid LOS	−4%	−4%	4%
% Chg. - Disp Shr Payment per MCR dischg.	105%	85%	105%

APPENDIX A

University-Based	Northeast	South	Midwest	West
126%	92%	137%	143%	128%
36%	42%	25%	42%	19%
38%	45%	32%	39%	19%
−1%	−7%	−3%	−1%	1%
73%	83%	80%	91%	73%
2%	56%	2%	−9%	−3%
−2%	4%	−7%	−6%	4%
53%	75%	51%	44%	46%
132%	183%	87%	162%	110%
1%	0%	−3%	3%	3%
−8%	−6%	−9%	−8%	−10%
−7%	−13%	−3%	−9%	0%
−11%	−17%	−8%	5%	−36%
−9%	−8%	−14%	−6%	−10%
0%	−2%	2%	−2%	−1%
−3%	−4%	0%	0%	−10%
19%				
28%	35%	18%	30%	27%
35%	28%	31%	42%	31%
36%	34%	33%	43%	27%
−18%	−17%	−13%	−24%	−14%
−31%	−37%	−27%	−32%	−29%
−6%	−19%	12%	−13%	0%
87%	119%	104%	73%	47%

TABLE A-6 Rate of Change in Activity by Top 50 Funding Criteria, 1990-2000

All Academic Health Centers, 2000
Percent Change 1990-2000
(bold values differ by p <.05)

Variable	Top 50, NIH, GME, DSH	Top 50, NIH and GME	Top 50, NIH and DSH
% Chg. - NIH Funding	120%	159%	123%
% Chg. - Total Residents—Hospital	40%	37%	5%
% Chg. - Residents per Bed	36%	39%	24%
% Chg. - GME $ per resident	5%	4%	−18%
% Chg. - Library Recurring Expense	82%	73%	78%
% Chg. - Nursing Graduates	16%	4%	0%
% Chg. - Average daily census	−6%	1%	−19%
% Chg. - Total ER visits	41%	90%	39%
% Chg. - Total outpatient visits	126%	200%	30%
% Chg. - Total Hospital Beds	4%	−1%	−12%
% Chg. - Occupancy Rate	−8%	−5%	−5%
% Chg. - Medicare IP Days—Total Hospital	−6%	−9%	−21%
% Chg. - Medicaid IP Days—Total Hospital	11%	−38%	−22%
% Chg. - Total IP Days—Hospital	−6%	−8%	−18%
% Chg. - % MCR IP Days (Hospital)	0%	−1%	−1%
% Chg. - % MCD IP Days (Hospital)	1%	**−9%**	**−2%**
% Chg. - Medicare Casemix Index	22%	21%	24%
% Chg. - FTE total personnel	29%	38%	−10%
% Chg. - FTE Nurses per 1000 IP Days	35%	39%	16%
% Chg. - Total FTE per 1000 IP Days	39%	36%	16%
% Chg. - Overall LOS	−18%	−22%	−16%
% Chg. - Medicare LOS	−32%	−28%	−29%
% Chg. - Medicaid LOS	7%	−19%	4%
% Chg. - Disp Shr Payment per MCR dischg.	101%	95%	48%

APPENDIX A

Top 50, GME and DSH	Top 50, NIH	Top 50, GME	Top 50, DSH	None
137%	120%	119%	166%	110%
34%	23%	22%	33%	36%
36%	23%	21%	25%	45%
−12%	−2%	−11%	−5%	−1%
78%	67%	86%	143%	62%
0%	−8%	11%	−2%	22%
−14%	7%	−7%	12%	−3%
53%	97%	53%	102%	26%
163%	236%	55%	166%	95%
−1%	4%	0%	11%	−5%
−7%	−9%	−6%	−8%	−11%
−8%	−7%	27%	16%	−16%
−9%	−14%	−21%	6%	−14%
−10%	−7%	−6%	−1%	−16%
0%	−1%	−2%	3%	0%
−1%	**−3%**	**−7%**	**1%**	**−3%**
10%	18%	16%	18%	23%
15%	46%	33%	29%	24%
34%	39%	52%	43%	26%
41%	40%	44%	20%	37%
−15%	−16%	−15%	−17%	−15%
−31%	−29%	−28%	−33%	−32%
−12%	0%	−14%	8%	−7%
147%	71%	100%	80%	81%

TABLE A-7 Comparison of Hospitals by Teaching Program Size, 2000

All Academic Health Centers, 2000
(bold values differ by p <.05)

Variable	AHC	Large Teaching	Small Teaching	Non-teaching, 100+ Beds
Total Residents—Hospital	**308**	**149**	**34**	N/M
Residents per Bed	**0.59**	**0.42**	**0.09**	N/M
GME $ per resident	**$65,200**	**$78,262**	**$72,599**	N/M
Average daily census	428	320	249	122
Total ER visits	57,690	54,408	44,516	25,862
Total outpatient visits	419,145	318,624	240,677	111,828
Total Hospital Beds	532	367	346	195
Occupancy Rate	**69%**	**66%**	**59%**	**46%**
Medicare IP Days—Total Hospital	40,331	33,959	32,294	15,592
Medicaid IP Days—Total Hospital	27,970	15,811	8,628	3,576
Total IP Days—Hospital	135,726	94,204	76,573	31,857
% MCR IP Days (Hospital)	**30%**	**37%**	**43%**	**52%**
% MCD IP Days (Hospital)	**20%**	**17%**	**11%**	**12%**
Medicare Casemix Index	**1.77**	**1.53**	**1.54**	**1.30**
FTE total personnel	3,774	2,566	1,895	812
FTE Nurses per 1,000 IP Days	6.8	6.8	6.1	5.6
Total FTE per 1,000 IP Days	**25.4**	**28.0**	**22.3**	**19.9**
Overall Length of Stay (LOS)	**5.8**	**5.3**	**4.9**	**4.6**
Medicare LOS	**6.5**	**6.5**	**5.9**	**5.5**
Medicaid LOS	**6.3**	**5.8**	**5.0**	**4.2**
DSH per Medicare dischg.	**$1,454**	**$1,081**	**$597**	**$457**
Has HIV/AIDS Unit	92%	79%	67%	38%
Has Burn Unit	57%	20%	23%	2%
Has Geriatric Unit	80%	73%	68%	48%
Has Neonatal Unit	83%	63%	57%	17%
Has Pediatric Unit	68%	44%	29%	6%
Has PET Scanner	48%	14%	17%	7%
Has Transplant Services	88%	26%	26%	5%
Has Trauma Center	87%	57%	57%	30%
Has Angioplasty center	96%	60%	72%	30%
Has Open Heart Surgery	95%	55%	67%	27%

* Small teaching means ACGME residency program or residents/bed >0.
* Nonteaching means any hospital not in the first three groups with 100+ beds in 2000.
** NM means not meaningful, because these hospitals have no residents.

TABLE A-8 Rate of Change in Activity by Teaching Program Size, 1990-2000

All Academic Health Centers, 2000
Percent Change, 1990-2000
(bold values differ by p <.05)

Variable	AHC	Large Teaching	Small Teaching*	Non-teaching, 100+ Beds*
% Chg. - Total Residents—Hospital	33%	26%	47%	NM**
% Chg. - Residents per Bed	35%	54%	61%	NM**
% Chg. - GME $ per resident	−3%	6%	11%	NM**
% Chg. - Average daily census	−2%	−18%	−6%	15%
% Chg. - Total ER visits	54%	35%	51%	45%
% Chg. - Total outpatient visits	133%	105%	138%	123%
% Chg. - Total Hospital Beds	0%	−16%	−9%	−6%
% Chg. - Occupancy Rate	−8%	−9%	−6%	−7%
% Chg. - Medicare IP Days—Total Hospital	−7%	−30%	−9%	−13%
% Chg. - Medicaid IP Days—Total Hospital	−10%	−2%	11%	13%
% Chg. - Total IP Days—Hospital	−10%	−25%	−5%	−16%
% Chg. - % MCR IP Days (Hospital)	0%	−4%	−2%	1%
% Chg. - % MCD IP Days (Hospital)	−2%	−1%	1%	1%
% Chg. - Medicare Casemix Index	20%	14%	11%	7%
% Chg. - FTE total personnel	26%	12%	30%	32%
% Chg. - FTE Nurses per 1,000 IP Days	33%	61%	45%	46%
% Chg. - Total FTE per 1,000 IP Days	35%	60%	46%	45%
% Chg. - Overall Length of Stay (LOS)	−17%	−25%	−22%	−19%
% Chg. - Medicare LOS	−31%	−35%	−31%	−27%
% Chg. - Medicaid LOS	−4%	−9%	−10%	−12%
% Chg. - DSH per Medicare dischg.	91%	92%	69%	72%

* Small teaching means ACGME residency program or residents/bed >0.
* Nonteaching means any hospital not in the first three groups with 100+ beds in 2000.
** NM means not meaningful, because these hospitals have no residents.

TABLE A-9 Provision of Specialized Serviced by Teaching Status

Provision of Specialized Services
Who Provides What Services

Variable	AHC	Large Teaching	Small Teaching	Nonteaching
Total Hospital Beds	10%	8%	31%	51%
Medicare Inpatient Days—Hospital	9%	9%	34%	48%
Medicaid Inpatient Days—Hospital	20%	17%	30%	34%
Total Inpatient Days—Hospital	13%	11%	35%	41%
Interns and Residents—Hospital	48%	30%	22%	0%
Total Medicare Discharges—Hospital	8%	8%	34%	50%
Total Medicaid Discharges—Hospital	16%	14%	30%	41%
Total Discharges—Hospital	11%	10%	35%	44%
Has HIV AIDS Unit	10%	8%	20%	62%
Has Burn Unit	43%	16%	17%	23%
Has Geriatrics Unit	6%	6%	16%	72%
Has Neonatal Unit	16%	12%	31%	41%
Has Pediatric Unit	23%	16%	29%	32%
Has >1 PET Scanner	22%	7%	23%	48%
Has Single PET Scanner	8%	5%	18%	69%
Has Transplant Services	33%	10%	28%	29%
Has Trauma Center	9%	6%	18%	67%
Has Angioplasty Center	13%	8%	29%	50%
Has Open Heart Surgery	15%	9%	32%	43%
Percent of Hospitals	3%	4%	9%	84%

SOURCES: Hospital Cost Report Information System, 1999; American Hospital Association, 2000.

TABLE A-10 IS ON THE NEXT PAGE

TABLE A-10 Comparison of Market Share by Teaching Program Size

Summary of Market Share for AHC and Other Hospitals
Hospital Cost Report Information System (HCRIS), 1990 and 1999
12-Month Reporting Period; Short Term, Non-Federal Hospitals

Hospital Cost Report Information System, 1990 (sums)	AHC	Large Teaching	Small Teaching	Nonteaching
Total Hospital Beds	63,492	46,357	278,088	480,139
Medicare Inpatient Days— Total Hospital	5,391,356	4,320,665	29,998,331	43,837,324
Medicaid Inpatient Days— Total Hospital	4,081,416	2,969,668	8,142,101	8,978,683
Total Inpatient Days—Hospital	18,126,428	13,220,641	67,855,270	88,833,843
Interns and Residents—Hospital	29,233	20,017	22,808	—
Total MCR Discharges—Hospital	557,916	430,066	3,289,418	5,602,497
Total MCD Discharges—Hospital	619,421	475,744	1,376,539	1,804,251
Total Discharges—Hospital	2,577,235	1,939,022	10,611,524	15,464,833
% of Hospitals	2%	2%	17%	79%
% of Totals				
Total Hospital Beds	7%	5%	32%	55%
Medicare Inpatient Days— Total Hospital	6%	5%	36%	52%
Medicaid Inpatient Days— Total Hospital	17%	12%	34%	37%
Total Inpatient Days—Hospital	10%	7%	36%	47%
Interns and Residents—Hospital	41%	28%	32%	0%
Total MCR Discharges—Hospital	6%	4%	33%	57%
Total MCD Discharges—Hospital	14%	11%	32%	42%
Total Discharges—Hospital	8%	6%	35%	51%

TABLE A-10 Continued

Hospital Cost Report Information System, 1999 (sums)				
Total Hospital Beds	63,064	52,395	198,408	321,031
Medicare Inpatient Days—Hospital	4,763,347	4,669,159	18,009,980	24,925,268
Medicaid Inpatient Days—Hospital	3,306,950	2,776,128	4,946,093	5,691,269
Total Inpatient Days— Hospital	16,050,935	13,689,631	43,257,039	50,686,618
Interns and Residents—Hospital	36,111	22,376	16,270	—
Total MCR Discharges—Hospital	724,861	698,953	2,998,947	4,510,503
Total MCD Discharges—Hospital	554,365	489,894	1,044,790	1,447,558
Total Discharges—Hospital	2,776,901	2,535,508	8,941,337	11,158,306
% of Hospitals	3%	4%	18%	75%
% of Totals				
Total Hospital Beds	10%	8%	31%	51%
Medicare Inpatient Days—Hospital	9%	9%	34%	48%
Medicaid Inpatient Days—Hospital	20%	17%	30%	34%
Total Inpatient Days—Hospital	13%	11%	35%	41%
Interns and Residents—Hospital	48%	30%	22%	0%
Total MCR Discharges—Hospital	8%	8%	34%	50%
Total MCD Discharges—Hospital	16%	14%	30%	41%
Total Discharges—Hospital	11%	10%	35%	44%

APPENDIX B

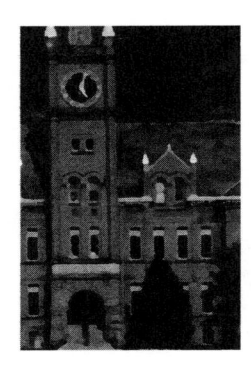

COMMITTEE ON THE ROLES OF ACADEMIC HEALTH CENTERS IN THE 21ST CENTURY

WORKSHOP ON THE ROLES OF ACADEMIC HEALTH CENTERS

Final Agenda
Melrose Hotel, 2430 Pennsylvania Ave., N.W.,
Washington, D.C.
January 24–25, 2002

Thursday, January 24

8:00   Continental breakfast available

8:30–8:40   Welcome, opening remarks
John Edward Porter

8:40–9:00   Introductions around the table

Section I: Changing Needs and Trends in Health Care

9:00–9:20   **How AHCs Can Meet the Future of Health Care**
Uwe E. Reinhardt, Ph.D., Professor of Economics and Public Affairs, Woodrow Wilson School of Public and International Affairs, Princeton University

APPENDIX B

9:20–9:40	**Future Trends and Directions in Health Care** Jeff Goldsmith, Ph.D., President, Health Futures, Inc. and Associate Professor of Medical Education, University of Virginia
9:40–10:00	Brief questions for Drs. Reinhardt and Goldsmith
10:00–10:30	**Changing Expectations for AHCs from Various Constituencies** • The Needs of Patients: Ellen Stovall, Executive Director, National Coalition for Cancer Survivorship • The Needs of Low-Income Populations: Sara Rosenbaum, J.D., Harold and Jane Hirsh Professor of Law and Policy, The George Washington University School of Public Health and Health Services • The Needs of Health Plans: Charles Cutler, M.D., Chief Medical Officer, American Association of Health Plans
10:30–11:10	Q&A for all morning presenters • Do different constituencies have conflicting expectations for AHCs? • Which trends and expectations are likely to have a particularly significant impact on the roles performed by AHCs?
11:10–11:20	Break

Section II: Creating a Vision for the Future

Panel on the Clinical Service Role

11:20–11:35	Peter Kohler, M.D., President, Oregon Health Sciences University
11:35–11:50	Ezra Davidson, M.D., Associate Dean, Charles R. Drew University of Medicine and Science
11:50–12:30	Questions for panelists and general discussion • As competition in clinical services grows and more sources of care are available, where does the AHC fit into the delivery system?

- To what extent is the academic relationship a differentiating factor in the marketplace?
- Do AHCs have a role in developing efficient and effective models of care for the populations dependent upon them?

12:30–1:15	Lunch/break
	Panel on the Education and Training Role
1:15–1:30	A Perspective from Medicine: Edward Hundert, M.D., Dean, University of Rochester School of Medicine and Dentistry
1:30–1:45	A Perspective from Nursing: Colleen Conway-Welch, Ph.D., R.N., Dean and Professor, School of Nursing, Vanderbilt University
1:45–2:00	A Perspective from Public Health: James W. Curran, M.D., M.P.H., Dean and Professor of Epidemiology, The Rollins School of Public Health, Emory University
2:00–2:45	Questions for panelists and general discussion

- How will training programs in medicine, nursing, and public health relate to each other to effectively train health professionals in the future? Can linkages be created among the medical, behavioral, and social sciences to improve health?
- Will education become more expensive in the future? Why?
- To what extent will changes in the education and training role impact the clinical service and/or research roles, or are the future changes in this role independent of other roles?

2:45–3:00	Break
	Panel on the Research Role
3:00–3:15	Biomedical Research: Gerald Fischbach, M.D., Executive Vice President for Health and Biomedical Sciences; Dean, Faculty of Health Sciences; Dean, Faculty of Medicine, Columbia University College of Physicians and Surgeons

APPENDIX B   201

3:15–3:30   Clinical Research: Ralph Snyderman, M.D., Chancellor
               for Health Affairs; Executive Dean, School of Medicine;
               President and CEO, Duke University Health System

3:30–3:45   Perspectives from Private Industry: Samuel Broder,
               M.D., Executive Vice President, Celera Genomics

3:45–4:00   Health Services Research: Ralph I. Horwitz, M.D., Yale
               University School of Medicine

4:00–4:45   Questions for panelists and general discussion
               • Are research relationships between AHCs and private
                 industry likely to increase or decrease in the future?
                 What are the potential benefits and concerns that arise
                 in research relationships between AHCs and private
                 industry?
               • How do AHCs set research priorities? Who has input
                 in defining priorities?
               • How important are concerns surrounding technology
                 transfer? What is the role of the university in
                 technology transfer?

4:45–5:00   Thanks to those leaving; committee's next steps; adjourn

Friday, January 25

8:00   Continental breakfast available

8:30–8:45   Call to order; announcements; new introductions
               John Edward Porter, Chair

               *Section III: Creating an Environment to Support
               Needed Changes*

8:45–9:10   **Critical Issues to Confront in Studying Academic Health
               Centers**
               David Blumenthal, M.D., Executive Director,
               Commonwealth Task Force on Academic Health
               Centers; Director, Institute for Health Policy,
               Massachusetts General Hospital/Partners HealthCare
               System, Inc.

9:10–9:40	Questions and Discussion
9:40–10:00	**Financial Issues Affecting the Future of Academic Health Centers** Bruce Vladeck, Ph.D., Senior Vice President for Policy, Mount Sinai/NYU Health
10:00–10:20	Questions and discussion
10:20–10:30	Break
10:30–10:50	**An AHC's View on Cross-Subsidies and the Implications for Shifting Priorities** Darrell G. Kirch, M.D., Senior Vice President for Health Affairs; Dean, College of Medicine; CEO, Penn State Milton S. Hershey Medical Center, Pennsylvania State University
10:50–11:10	Questions and discussion
11:10–11:30	**Variation in the Roles Pursued by Academic Health Centers** Gerard F. Anderson, Ph.D., Professor and Director, Center for Hospital Finance and Management, The Johns Hopkins University Bloomberg School of Public Health
11:30–11:50	Questions and discussion
11:50–12:15	General Discussion • Are all AHCs affected equally by the changing trends? Are all AHCs equally prepared to meet changing community needs? • To what extent can AHCs make changes desired by both themselves and their communities within current financing methods (e.g., if more ambulatory and multidisciplinary education is desired, can it be done)? • What are the *nonfinancially* related needs of AHCs to adapt to a changing health system?
12:15	Committee's next steps; thanks; adjourn John Edward Porter, Chair